From Apprenticeship to Graduate Pharmacy Programmes

From Apprenticeship to Graduate Pharmacy Programmes

Evolution of Pharmacy Education in Jamaica

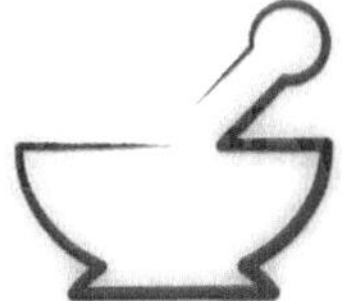

Eugenie Brown-Myrie &
Yvonne Johnson-Reid

University of Technology, Jamaica Press

First published in Jamaica 2021 by
University of Technology, Jamaica Press
237 Old Hope Road
Kingston 6
Email: utechjapress@utech.edu.jm

A catalogue record of this book is available from the
National Library of Jamaica.

ISBN: 978-976-96211-2-1 (print)
978-976-96211-4-5 (Kindle)

Cover and book design by Robert Harris
Email: roberth@cwjamaica.com

Set in Minion Pro 11.5/16 x 27

Printed in the USA.

Contents

APPENDICES

List of Illustrations

Foreword

This is an excellent book which looks at the knowledge about the Pharmaceutical education and practice systems retrospectively and prospectively. The two authors of this excellent book, Eugenie Brown-Myrie and Yvonne Johnson-Reid, have straddled in real time, some of the years of this documented history, not only as students but also as practitioners who can speak with clarity and also authority (as noted in the book).

Some of the highlights of this book, are the stories of apprenticeship for pharmacists prior to the training programme at the College of Arts, Science & Technology (CAST). This period for those who are aware was a period when pharmacy was truly "an art and a science" combined. This is based on the elegant compounding and preparation of which these pharmacists prepared and dispensed with grace and outstanding professionalism. In my view this represents the golden age of pharmacy.

During this time, there were people like Dick Kinkead, who transcended that golden period into the era of modern pharmacy. I can attest to this through the constant research and development of new pharmaceuticals particularly, from plant origins. For example, after I became acquainted with Dick, he got the idea of looking at the development of what he called the "Jamaican toothpaste." We developed a new toothpaste called "Chewdent" which only disappeared from the shelves after approximately 30 years. The sad thing is that most innovations like this one, have not received the necessary support and recognition, either through lack of information or negligence.

For me, the next most important era was the transitional training of the pharmacist at CAST in which I was fully involved. This was such a stimulant for me that I decided to find a specialist area in pharmacy to make my special contribution. My dream was realized when I obtained a Commonwealth Scholarship to Sydney University in Australia, where I pursued the Master of Science in Pharmaceutical/Medicinal Chemistry, which was at that time a new and emerging area of pharmacy being developed to meet the requirement of the new era of pharmacy. In addition, in consideration of succession planning, it was necessary to have a replacement for Mr Bernard Towlson, lecturer in pharmaceutical chemistry. While being an outstanding lecturer, as an English man, he was due to return home within a couple of years. It was my intention to succeed him and ensure that this area of pharmacy education had continuity.

During this time, I encouraged and mentored Carol White and George Roper who were my successors. George Roper moved up the Administration ladders to assume the role as Vice Principal with responsibility for Academic Affairs and Research. I can also recall the influence of senior pharmacists such as Vin Bennett and Lester Woolery, who played a major role in the development of pharmacy in Jamaica. I can also remember the contributions of enthusiastic pharmacy students towards the development of pharmacy education while I was Head of the Science Department. One of the most significant achievements was the building out of the undercroft, a section of the Science building for a library and a classroom since the resources were limited at that time. Then there was the era of bright enterprising students such as Grace Allen-Young and Eugenie Brown-Myrie, and others who not only demonstrated the quality of the education but also their own abilities by going overseas and competing in the international academic arena and returning to Jamaica to give outstanding leadership in pharmacy education and practice.

Perhaps one of the greatest achievements was the recognition of our graduates and the acceptance to academic programmes and institutions in North America and Europe. For me, the greatest achievement was the negotiations with Professor Ron Scott, Dean of Pharmacy at Howard

University. CAST students were accepted and afforded advanced status and scholarships to pursue the Bachelor of Pharmacy (BPharm) degree. I recall the personal contributions of Dr Hugh Lunan and Dr Yvonne Crichton, Jamaicans who having been trained at the doctoral level returned to Jamaica to make sacrificial contribution to the modernization of the pharmacy programme at CAST.

Today I am not only delighted, but proud to see the progression in the growth and development of a pharmacy programme, from humble beginnings to the noble heights of a graduate Doctor of Pharmacy programme which we have accomplished, not only for the benefit of Jamaica but the wider Caribbean. My question at this time, however, is whether the UWI pharmacy degree programme could have been dovetailed with the training programme at UTech, Jamaica to produce a more efficient and effective programme for the Caribbean region.

I proudly associate myself with this manuscript because of the positive history and perspective which it offers for the future. This book should not only be purchased by every pharmacist in Jamaica but should be required textbook for all pharmacy students across the Caribbean region. Once again, I congratulate the authors of this book Eugenie Brown-Myrie and Yvonne Johnson-Reid and wish them well. I thank them for granting me the opportunity to be associated with this outstanding publication.

Professor the Hon. Henry I.C. Lowe, O.J., CD., J.P., PhD. (Man), DSc. (Hons.), F.R.S.H. (UK)
Executive Chairman, Environmental Health Foundation | R&D Group of Companies

Preface

The Caribbean suffers from a dearth of publications and general information that address issues and situations unique to the region. Despite the fact that the landscape is changing, it is very difficult to find information on specific matters relating to health and education. The authors were concerned that they could not find documented information relating to Pharmacy Education and Training despite the fact that training of pharmacists has been conducted locally since the late nineteenth century. The University of Technology, Jamaica, (formerly, the College of Arts, Science and Technology [CAST]), has delivered pharmacy education for more than fifty years (57 years, in 2019).

The book documents the various approaches and formats used to deliver pharmacy education and training in Jamaica for a period which spanned over 100 years. The time period has been divided into different eras to highlight the evolution of the training. The book also outlines how the training over the review period reflected modifications in an effort to address the dynamic changes in the professional and practice environments. The book highlights the educational approaches utilized in an effort to meet international academic standards.

Pharmacy education initiatives in Jamaica are recorded in a chronological way. The book provides useful information on the subject matter and creates an avenue for review and future expansion of the work in this academic area.

The book chronicles the historical evolution of the education and training of pharmacists in Jamaica from the late nineteenth century to the present. It documents details of the period of training which started under an apprenticeship regime to the formalized, institutionalized programme delivery at the University of Technology, Jamaica, in 1962.

This long over-due publication will serve to inform and create awareness among the members of the pharmacy profession. It will also serve as a textbook for students enrolled in the Pharmacy discipline. Through this publication, the students will learn about the progress made in the evolution of pharmacy education in Jamaica. It is expected that the publication will serve to motivate and instill pride in the members of the pharmacy fraternity. Additionally, it should help to motivate and encourage persons who may wish to contribute to the body of knowledge about aspects of the education of pharmacy professionals.

In 2016, the University of the West Indies implemented the first Entry Level Doctor of Pharmacy degree programme and has joined the ranks as an approved institution for the training of pharmacists. Jamaica has played a pivotal role in the offering of pharmacy education locally and regionally, as the University of Technology, Jamaica was the first academic institution to offer institutionalized education for pharmacists in the Caribbean. This contribution to pharmacy education has continued for more than a half century. Much of the information about the history of pharmacy education was obtained by word of mouth as prior to this date, very little had been documented about pharmacy education in the region.

Since very little had been written formally, the authors sought to record aspects of the history drawn from their academic work and professional experiences and involvement relating to pharmacy education. Additional information was obtained from other sources, including interviews, personal communications, writings of other colleagues, and several pharmacy publications. The intent is to preserve this legacy of pharmacy education in Jamaica.

Acknowledgments

This publication would not have been possible without the written presentations of several pharmacy stalwarts who recorded valuable information about training and practice of pharmacy in Jamaica. Among this group of pioneers are, Leo Vaughn, Lester Woolery, Grace Allen-Young and Ellen Campbell-Grizzle. A significant amount of information was retrieved from the Caribbean Pharmacy News Series, a publication edited by Dr Ellen Campbell-Grizzle over a period of approximately six years. Other publications which served as valuable sources of information were the *PCJ Updates*, a publication of the Pharmacy Council of Jamaica, Pharmaceutical Society of Jamaica magazines, Minutes of meetings and conferences and Reports presented at conferences.

The authors must also recognize Dr Alfred Sangster, former President of UTech, Jamaica who has been a source of inspiration over their professional and academic years, but more importantly, for his book, titled, *"The Making of a University: From CAST to UTech, 2010"* which served as an important point of reference for this publication.

Special recognition to Dr Ellen Campbell-Grizzle for her literary work through the *Pharmacy News* and *Periwinkle Papers*, which were documents cited by the authors in many sections of this volume. Those publications were the source of a wide range of valuable information.

We also wish to thank persons who shared their knowledge and experiences by way of interviews and notes.

Appreciation also goes to Dr Mearle Barrett, who reviewed the book and provided useful comments, which helped the authors to improve on the quality of the publication.

We acknowledge the contribution of Miss Keisha Dacres, who provided valuable administrative support for the project.

Recognition also goes to the pharmacy leaders who made tremendous sacrifices, developing policies and standards to guide the professional and academic strategies and decisions. We commend their professional and academic leadership.

Thanks to UTech, Jamaica Press for the financial and production support that made this publication possible.

Introduction

Pharmacy is among the oldest health professions practiced in Jamaica. Early information states that the practice of pharmacy in Jamaica began in the 1880s. At that time, the training was delivered through an apprenticeship system, which saw student pharmacists apprenticed to medical doctors who taught them what it was thought that the pharmacist then needed to know. This was mainly the practical aspect of dispensing – compounding, powder making, and the simpler features of making mixtures and ointments. It is assumed that this method of teaching, which was practiced in 19th century Europe, was transferred to this colony as well. (Reid, 2013)

The pharmacist was in those early days called "Doc" or "the Druggist" or "Dispenser," was almost always a man, and enjoyed a high level of respect from most citizens. Unfortunately, although the relationships between Doctors and Dispensers were usually cordial, the Dispenser was often seen as a 'left back' doctor who merely executed the will of the doctor, tried to interpret the doctor's prescriptions (which were often written in Latin) and practiced his skill of attending to minor ailments (Reid, 2013)

In those early days also, most doctors dispensed their own prescriptions. However, as training and opportunities increased for the Dispensers, many of them became owners/operators of retail and wholesale businesses called "Drug Stores". Among these establishments, Kinkead's in Kingston, Clementson & Tomlinson in St Mary, and Hylton & Hylton in Montego Bay stand out. Other large distributorships like Gideon & Gideon employed their own Dispensers (Reid, 2013).

As the trade in pharmaceuticals grew, some of the larger "drug stores" became importers and representatives of overseas pharmaceutical companies. Between 1930 and 1950, many new pharmaceutical products were developed overseas and introduced to the Jamaican market. This led to an influx of products from new pharmaceutical companies into the island. At this time also, pressure from various sources led to many doctors ceasing the practice of 'dispensing'. This opened even more avenues for enterprising Dispensers.

As medical knowledge became more available to the populace, greater reliance was placed in manufactured pharmaceuticals, and less on traditional 'home remedies' so that by the 1950s, retail pharmacies were well established in the Kingston and St Andrew metropolitan area. Its spread to the rural areas was slower.

Acronyms & Abbreviations

AAIMS	American Allied International Medical School
ACPE	Accreditation Council for Pharmacy Education
ALCOA	Aluminum Company of America
ASHP	American Society of Health Systems Pharmacists
AY	Academic Year
BP	British Pharmacopoeia
CAAM-HP	Caribbean Accreditation Agency for Medicine and other Health Professions
CARPIN	Caribbean Poison Information Network
CAP	Caribbean Association of Pharmacists
CAPE	Caribbean Advanced Proficiency Examination
CPA	Commonwealth Pharmacists Association
CARICOM	Caribbean Community
CAST	College of Arts, Science and Technology
CCAPP	Canadian Council for Accreditation of Pharmacy Programs
CE	Continuing Education
CET	Continuing Education and Training
CIDA	Canadian International Development Agency
CIPPPAR	Caribbean Institute of Pharmacy Policy, Practice and Research

COB	College of the Bahamas
CPD	Continuing Professional Development
CPhA	Canadian Pharmaceutical Association
CPhT	Certified Pharmacy Technician
CPN	Caribbean Pharmacy News
CSEC	Caribbean Secondary Examination Council
CSHP	Canadian Society of Hospital Pharmacists
CXC	Caribbean Examination Council
EQA	External Quality Assurance
FDA	Food and Drug Administration
FIP	International Pharmaceutical Federation
GICS	Global Institute of Certified Specialists
GCE	General Certificate of Education
HECOIN	Health Education and Counseling Institute
HIV/AIDs	Human Immunodeficiency Virus/Acquired Immunodeficiency Disease
IPSF	International Pharmaceutical Students Federation
KPH	Kingston Public Hospital
MFPI	Manual for Pharmacy Internship
MPhil	Master of Philosophy
MOH	Ministry of Health
MOHEC	Ministry of Health and Environmental Control
NGO	Non-Governmental Organisation
NHF	National Health Fund
NTPD	Non-Traditional PharmD
PAHO	Pan American Health Organisation
PCJ	Petroleum Corporation of Jamaica
PCJ	Pharmacy Council of Jamaica

PACE	Pharmacy and Apotex Continuing Education
PHACE	Pharmacists Active in Continuing Education
PharmD	Doctor of Pharmacy
PhD	Doctor of Philosophy
PSJ	Pharmaceutical Society of Jamaica
PTCB	Pharmacy Technician Certification Board
UHWI	University Hospital of the West Indies
UF	University of Florida
UK	United Kingdom
UOD	University of Derby
UWI	University of the West Indies
WHO	World Health Organisation
UCJ	University Council of Jamaica
UTech, Jamaica	University of Technology, Jamaica

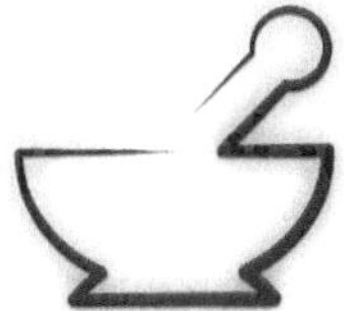

1.

Pre-Institutionalization

The beginning and evolution of pharmacy education and training in Jamaica progressed through several phases or eras. This book will define two main levels of training: undergraduate and graduate. Each level will be further discussed according to the various era or stage of development.

UNDERGRADUATE EDUCATION AND TRAINING

Pre-KPH Era

Prior to the twentieth (20th) century, pharmacy practice was very informal and lacked proper standards. The training of Pharmacists, then called Dispensers, was through the apprenticeship system which had become very widespread in the latter part of the nineteenth century. Pharmacists understudied doctors and it is significant to note that pharmacists trained after the Emancipation and before the 1900s were entitled to practice medicine.

By the 1890s, it became evident that formalised pharmacy education was a necessity. At that time, there were already institutions in the United States of America, e.g. Philadelphia College of Pharmacy and Science and the University of Manchester in Great Britain where formal pharmacy training was offered (Remington, 2012). The Victoria University in Great Britain was the first University to offer an honours degree in pharmacy in 1904. Victoria University went on to become one of the two institutions that formed the new University of Manchester in 2004. (https://www.bmh.manchester.ac.uk/about/history-heritage.)

According to Lowe (1973), pharmacy education in Jamaica was formalized in 1890 with training conducted either at the Kingston Public Hospital or a Doctor's surgery. In those days the entry requirement was English Language, Arithmetic, General Studies and Latin. The curriculum was designed to produce professional "Druggists" who would be proficient in the areas of compounding, dispensing, prescription writing, therapeutics, drug incompatibilities and Materia Medica and a thorough knowledge of the British Pharmacopeia. An early Graduate, Pharmacist Paula Ellis in an interview corroborated the information on training as she informed the interviewer that students who did not leave to study in a foreign school were trained at Kingston Public Hospital (then called "Chocho Gully", or at a Medical Doctor's surgery.

In those days, a theory examination was set by the Chief Medical Officer (KPH) and the practical examination was set by the Chief Druggist. On successful completion of the course, a Certificate and a Licence to practice as a Druggist were awarded (Lowe, 1973). The programme equipped the Druggist to function with, and in many cases for the doctor, and was often called "Doc".

Lowe further posited that several changes in entry requirement and curriculum took place during 1940 and 1960 at the KPH. Some of these included the replacement of Arithmetic with Mathematics and the inclusion of a Science subject. More attention was given to didactic training, with the expansion of the Pharmacology and Organic Chemistry disciplines. Additionally, the role of the "Druggist" began to change to involve more compounding and dispensing services and far less clinical services. He opined that the leaders of the Pharmacy profession, the Ministry of Health and the Government of Jamaica of the day recognised that the training of professional pharmacists required institutionalised training, with modern approaches to teaching and a much broader curriculum to adequately satisfy the new demands of the profession and practice. As a result, the Pharmacy Department was established at the College of Arts, Science and Technology (CAST), Jamaica in 1961 (Lowe, 1973).

The KPH/ Pre-CAST Era

The training of pharmacists (Druggists) at the Kingston Public Hospital officially began in 1911 and continued until 1964 (Reid, 2013). By the 1920s the entry requirements for study of "*dispensing*", as it was called, was a Senior Cambridge School Certificate based on an examination set by the University of Cambridge, UK. The academic requirements to matriculate into the pharmacy training during that dispensation was English Language, Arithmetic, General Studies and Latin, the latter being desirable but was not compulsory. The course of study was geared to produce druggists proficient in dispensing, compounding, prescription writing, therapeutics, drug incompatibilities, the Materia Medica and a thorough knowledge of the British Pharmacopeia, B.P. (Reid, 2013).

The three-year course of study incorporated such subjects as Simple Dentistry (mainly extractions), Administration of Parenterals and Anaesthetics, Surgical Dressing Applications, Medical Record Keeping, Operating Theatre Procedures, Venereal Disease Control, Medical Stores Management, Financial Controlling, and the Preparation of Death Certificates and other Legal documents. There were courses that entailed the actual **feeling, smelling and tasting** of various pharmaceutical products so that the Dispenser could fully "identify drugs" (Reid, 2013).

An Externship took the form of weekly working visits – along with a medical doctor – to outlying clinics (called "Out-stations"). At the end of the three-year course, students sat an examination which was spread over 2–3 days. The practical was examined by the Chief Dispenser/Druggist and theory aspects examined by the Senior Medical Officer. Those who passed the exams were awarded a Certificate, which authorized them to become licensed to practice as a Dispenser or more specifically "to sell Drugs and Poisons (Robertson, 2016).

The 1940–1960s saw some adjustments to the matriculation requirements to enter the KPH course. Although the same three passes in the Senior Cambridge School Certificate was a requirement, Latin could determine one's entry into the course. Curriculum changes included a greater emphasis on didactic needs and the introduction of more pharmacology and organic chemistry in the course. The pharmacist's role also began to change to reflect a greater involvement in compounding and dispensing services and provision of less clinical services (Lowe, 1973).

The authors' research revealed a copy of a Certification Letter for a graduate of the 3-year course of Study at the end of the KPH era (Appendix 1). The document showed that students had to sit and pass five subjects in order to be awarded the Druggist's Licence. In 1962, those subjects were recorded as: Pharmaceutical Chemistry, Pharmaceutics and Materia Medica, Forensic Pharmacy, Practical Dispensing and Identifications and Orals. The Pass Mark for each subject and the course from those early days was set at 60 per cent.

The education and training were broad-based, producing a multi-skilled practitioner. This early training of pharmacists equipped them to function in many practice areas designed for the doctor, such as, giving anesthetics and setting bones. Graduates of the programme of study also 'advanced' to become Administrators, known as Hospital Secretaries, and Managers of Hospital Regions (Robertson, 2016).

The apprenticeship training had obvious inadequacies and disadvantages. It offered limited knowledge in the pure and applied sciences and the apprenticeship system was very onerous on the students as it afforded little time for study. These deficiencies became the propelling force for the implementation of a formalized course of study offered in an academic institution (Lowe, 1973).

The authors assume that persons trained between 1952 and 1965 were registered by the Drugs and Poisons Control Board under the Drugs and

Poisons Law, 1952. It is unclear what authority regulated the training of druggists prior to 1952. However, according to Gray and Woolery (2005), the Drugs and Poisons Law, was the Authority under which pharmacists were registered in 1936 (*PSJ Retreat Magazine*, 2005). The Pharmacy Act of 1966 repealed the Drugs and Poisons Law. The Pharmacy Act was promulgated in 1975, with the attendant Pharmacy Regulations, being gazetted in the same year.

Up until 1962, when the training of pharmacists was institutionalized, KPH was the only local training institution for pharmacists. After the training of pharmacists started at CAST (now, UTech, Jamaica), in 1962, the first batch of graduating students did their internship at Kingston Public Hospital and University Hospital of the West Indies pharmacies, where they were exposed to the practical applications of pharmacy. KPH therefore continued as a training site for the profession. Historical records reveal that the hospital and pharmacy department were very instrumental in convening international conferences and establishing links with overseas universities, such as University of London for student exchange. This allowed students to have opportunities for international exposure (Hall, 2003).

2.

Pharmacy Technicians and Assistants

PHARMACY TECHNICIAN TRAINING

Pharmacy technicians are trained pharmacy personnel who assist licensed pharmacists in the provision of pharmacy services to patients. They perform routine tasks to assist in dispensing prescribed medications such as counting tablets, weighing and measuring pharmaceutical ingredients and labeling preparations and proprietary products. Their roles may extend to maintaining patient profiles, preparing insurance claims, maintaining pharmacy inventory and selling over the counter medications. They work at all times under the supervision of a licensed pharmacist.

Formal pharmacy technician education and training programmes involve classroom and laboratory work in a variety of areas, including medical and pharmaceutical terminology, pharmaceutical calculations, pharmacy recordkeeping, pharmacy law and ethics. They are also exposed to medication names, actions, uses, and doses. Many training programmes include an internship component during which students gain hands on experience in actual pharmacies. Students receive a diploma, certificate or an associate degree at graduation, depending on the programme.

UK Training

One of the authors (Reid, 2018) reminisced on her first encounter with Mrs Lillith Squire, whom she met in 1972 when she gained practical experience at the Pharmacy Department of the Kingston Public Hospital as a pharmacy student. She described Mrs Squire as a very pleasant lady; always wearing a smile. Mrs Squire was introduced as a Pharmacy Technician trained in England.

On Wednesday, February 28, 2018, during a telephone interview, Mrs Squire related that she was trained in UK during the period 1961–1963. She was trained at London College for Pharmacy and Chemists for Women in the United Kingdom. The didactic training was for one year and this was followed by one-year of internship at St. Giles Hospital, Camberwell South East. She reported that she worked in the areas of Medical Practice and Veterinary Surgery. She received certification as a Dispenser and worked at Giles Hospital until 1967, prior to returning home to Jamaica in November 1967. She explained that prior to her return to Jamaica the school in the UK closed and later reopened to train Pharmacy Technicians. By then, the degree for pharmacists was being offered in Pharmacy Schools in the UK and practitioners bore the designation of "Pharmacist."

On her return to Jamaica, she was advised that she needed to go to the College of Arts, Science and Technology (now, UTech, Jamaica) for 1 year in order to be licensed to practice as a pharmacist in Jamaica. For economic reasons she opted to seek employment and worked under the designation of Pharmacy Technician. She worked for 2 years at the Pharmacy Department of the Bustamante Hospital for Children, starting February 1968, then on to the Kingston Public Hospital Pharmacy Department in November 1970, where she continued until her retirement.

Hope Ship

Training for Pharmacy Technicians began under the Project HOPE (a People to People Health Foundation, Inc., Washington, D.C.) course of study in the early 1970s. This training was undertaken by the Ministry of Health and Environmental Control (MOHEC). The Director of Pharmaceutical Services at the time was Mr Lester Woolery. Mr George W. Strein, Jr., a pharmacist serving Project HOPE assumed the position on the committee for Pharmacy Technician Training for the MOHEC in Jamaica. Pharmacy Technicians served primarily as support staff for pharmacists in the public sector. As graduate pharmacists became more involved in clinical and teaching roles, (especially in hospitals) the need for support staff increased.

Ministry of Health Training

The Ministry of Health's involvement in Pharmacy Technician Training followed the Project HOPE programme in the mid-1970s. The training continued up to 1992. Telephone interview with Miss Roxanne Brown, Pharmacy Technician trained during 1990–1991 provided the following information. The training was for a period of one calendar year, divided into eight months of didactic education, delivered at the Glen Vincent Polyclinic and four months practical at the Comprehensive Health Centre (Type 5 Clinic) and the Bellevue Hospital, a specialist psychiatric hospital. From her recollection, persons who provided instruction in the programme were Mr Granville Forbes, Mrs Margaret Wilson-Blake, pharmacists at the University Hospital of the West Indies, and an elderly lady of Indian descent, whose name she does not recall but who might have been the Coordinator. She was awarded a Certificate on completion of the training. Miss Brown was in the second to last batch of students trained by the Ministry of Health. For a period of seven years (1992–1999), the formal training of Pharmacy Technicians in Jamaica ceased.

University Hospital of the West Indies Training Programme

The Education Unit of the University Hospital Pharmacy began training of Pharmacy Technicians in 1999. Candidates wanting to enroll in the UHWI training programme were required to have 3 GCE O' Level subjects with passes A, B and C or in the CXC General Proficiency exam, I or II and III in English Language, Mathematics and Chemistry. An interview was also a part of the selection process and that might also include Proficiency tests in English and Mathematics. The one-year course of study was divided into six months didactic and six months vocational training. The programme comprised approximately 600 hours of learning opportunities, including personal development seminars and a Research Assignment. Graduates were presented with a Certificate on successful completion of the training (UHWI Pharmacy Technician Curriculum, 1999).

The first Coordinator for the Technician Training programme at UHWI was Mrs Margaret Wilson-Blake. Some instructors on the programme over the years were Mr Lester Woolery, Mrs Yvonne Johnson-Reid, Mrs Valerie Germaine, Mrs Margaret Wilson-Blake and Mrs Julie-Ann Robinson-Jemmott. Graduates of this UHWI programme were equipped to work in both public and private sector pharmacies.

University of Technology, Jamaica Pharmacy Technician Training Programme

In academic year 2009/10, The University of Technology, Jamaica embarked on the training of Pharmacy Technicians in collaboration with the Ministry of Health as a Project. The academic year 2012/13 brought an end to the MOH/UTech, Jamaica's collaboration and UTech, Jamaica assumed full responsibility for the Technician's training. The course was delivered on a full-time basis over a calendar year for the first three cohorts. The restructured course of study is now delivered part-time over 18 months. This affords individuals the opportunity to study evenings and Saturdays without giving up their jobs. On successful completion, students receive a Certificate. The first Programme Director for the Pharmacy Technicians trained under the UTech, Jamaica curriculum was Mrs Yvonne Johnson-Reid.

Duly Certified Pharmacy Technicians are now advocating for UTech,

Jamaica to offer a higher level of training to the Associate degree as well as other specialties (Reid, 2013).

Other Providers of Pharmacy Technician Training

In addition to UTech, Jamaica's involvement in the training of Pharmacy Technicians, several private agencies are now offering training in Jamaica. Among them are: American Allied International Medical School (AAIMS), Health Education & Counseling Institute (HECOIN), Distinction College, and Global Institute of Certified Specialists (GICS). Some Pharmacy Technicians access training through online overseas programmes such as the Penn Foster Career School.

Apprenticeship Training – An ongoing situation

The training of Pharmacy Technicians under an apprenticeship system might have existed prior to the Hope Ship programme and continues to the present time. Currently, several community pharmacy technicians still obtain their training on the job. Unfortunately, these technicians do not have official certification. With the impending Registration of Pharmacy Technicians by the Pharmacy Council of Jamaica, Pharmacy Technicians may then be required to obtain official Certification after sitting and passing a Certification examination.

Pharmacy Assistant Training

The Education Unit at the UHWI Pharmacy started a Pharmacy Assistant Training Course in the year 2000 as an on the job training programme to equip staff employed to the institution. UTech, Jamaica commenced training of Pharmacy Assistants in June 2014. This short course for Pharmacy Assistants was delivered over a six-week period; 15 hours / week. The curriculum focused primarily on Communication and Non-prescription Drugs.

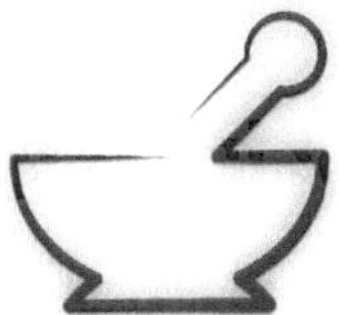

3.

Institutionalization

Diploma in Pharmacy

Institutionalised pharmacy training was established at the College of Arts, Science and Technology in 1962 as a three-year full-time Diploma in Pharmacy. Stafford Haughton recalls his first day in the programme at CAST. He recounted, "our first day was on January 06, 1962. I was accepted for the first batch of some 13 or 14 students to be trained as pharmacists to the Diploma level in a formal College environment." According to Haughton (2018), the Department of Pharmacy was fully integrated into the Faculty of Science. Sangster (2010) recorded that the Pharmacy Diploma was the first full-time course, to be introduced into the Science Department at the College. The introduction of the programme at CAST represented the first movement of a professional programme, which had previously been delivered by an apprenticeship system, to an academic institution.

The period 1963–4, marked the last batch of students to be trained at the Kingston Public Hospitals Pharmacy Department. The establishment of the Diploma in Pharmacy at the College of Arts Science and Technology (CAST) was realized through the strenuous collaborative efforts of The Ministry of Health (MOH), the Pharmaceutical Society of Jamaica (PSJ), the Ministry of Education and the relevant authorities at CAST (Sangster, 2010). The didactic training was followed by a period of six months internship. Although the first batch of students was a small number, it later increased to thirty per year (Sangster, 2010). The personal recollection of a graduate of the first batch of students, Stafford Haughton (2018) shared that there were ten students in the first class trained at CAST. There were five males, Stephen Jones, George Shim, Alfred Tenn, Vincent Bennett Jr and Stafford Haughton. There were five females, namely, Joan Melbourne-Neill, Molly Haynes, Joy Grant-Charles (withdrew at the end of the second year), Joan Thomas, and Dahlia Foster. All ten members of the pioneer group of pharmacists are still living and some still practice the Art of Pharmacy.

Graduates of the CAST course of study were awarded the Diploma in Pharmacy. The institution continued to produce Diploma in Pharmacy (Dip. Pharm) graduates for thirty-six years. The Diploma Programme was phased out thereafter. The last cohort of Diploma students was accepted into the College of Arts, Science and Technology in 1995.

Applicants entering the CAST Programme were required to matriculate with English Language, Mathematics and a Natural Science subject at the Senior Cambridge School Certificate Examination level. In later years, the qualifying examination was changed to the General Certificate Examination (GCE), at the Ordinary Level (O' Level), an examination originating at the University of Cambridge, in the United Kingdom. The General Certificate Examination (GCE), at the Ordinary Level (O' Level), replaced the Senior Cambridge Certificate.

The objectives of the curriculum were to: 1) provide an adequate background in the natural sciences and English required for the professional courses; 2) offer the necessary theoretical background and professional skill for later practice and 3) provide a balance between the theory and practice of pharmacy.

The Diploma programme was offered over two and a half years with

8 months internship post didactic education. During the first year, emphasis was placed on English and General Studies, Physics, Chemistry, Zoology and Botany. Year two focused on Dispensing, Pharmaceutics, Pharmacognosy, Organic Chemistry, Pharmaceutical Chemistry, and Physiology/Biochemistry. The final year concentrated on the expansion and introduction of new professional courses, such as, Dispensing, Pharmaceutics, Pharmacology, Organic Chemistry, Pharmaceutical Chemistry, Physiology, Pharmacognosy and Forensic Pharmacy.

At the end of the second year, during the summer period, a two-month period of vocational training was completed. Year 3 comprised six months of didactic training and an additional six-month vocational training (internship). A Diploma was awarded on the successful completion of the course at the College of Arts Science & Technology and a license granted by the Drugs and Poisons Control Board after the vocational training (Lowe, 1972). Since the inception of the Diploma in Pharmacy Programme, there have been a large number of changes to the curriculum, under the guidance of a Programme Advisory Committee.

With the establishment of the Pharmacy Council in 1966, the license to practice Pharmacy was granted by the Drugs and Poisons Board after successful completion of the 3 years training programme at CAST.

Pharmacists who completed the programme were equipped to meet the needs of the Jamaican patient, rendering services comparable to those of more developed countries in terms of delivery of health care.

The CAST-Howard University Initiative

Some changes were introduced in the 1973–1977 period to facilitate a CAST-Howard University collaboration which resulted in the award of a Bachelor of Science degree in Pharmacy. CAST students were afforded advanced placement in the Howard programme, where they completed one calendar year of instruction (Sangster 2010). On return to Jamaica, an additional 3–6 months of education was completed. The degree was then awarded by Howard University "in absentia."

The revisions to the programme included an increase in number of hours for professional subjects to create a better balance between professional and non-professional content of the programme. A primary objective was to meet matriculation requirement for entry into the CAST-Howard programme. Course changes included an expansion to the Organic Chemistry and Pharmacology syllabi, and the introduction of new courses such as, Socio-psychology, Therapeutics & Patient Care and Clinic Duty, as well as Pharmacy Administration.

Additional changes were introduced in the 1984–1988 period with several new courses being incorporated. Among them were Biostatistics, Technical Report Writing (Research Methods), Medical Terminology and Ethics, Immunology, Professional Practice and Computer Fundamentals. Nineteen eighty-eight (1988), also saw an increase in student intake from the usual thirty to fifty, in an effort to satisfy the increased demand for pharmacists.

Between 1989 and 1990, the Pharmacy curriculum was further restructured. The years 1 and 2 curriculum was modified to minimize content overlaps in course areas and also to reduce contact hours. Some courses were scheduled earlier in the programme. One such course was Pharmacology, which was advanced to year 2. Other School of Pharmacy achievements in that period were the establishment of a Drug Information Centre to support lecturers and students in the Pharmacy Diploma programme and a greater input from the Department in the Pharmacy Internship programme.

The changes in the Diploma of Pharmacy programmes were occurring at the same time that the Science Department was actively seeking to secure funds for the implementation of the Summer Modular Multidisciplinary Bachelor of Health Science Degree Programme. This Multidisciplinary Bachelor of Health Science offering would incorporate graduates from CAST Health Science Diploma Programmes and graduates of non-CAST equivalent level training programmes. The acquisition of funding from the W.K. Kellogg Foundation made the dream of the degree programme a reality in 1989 (Roper, 1990).

The Multi-Disciplinary Bachelor of Health Science Degree

In 1989, further progress was made in the educational aspect of the pharmacy profession as a Bachelor of Health Science Degree with a pharmacy specialization was introduced at the College of Arts, Science and Technology (CAST). The course of study was facilitated through a Kellogg Foundation Project grant to CAST to build the infrastructure for a Health Sciences Division and establish a degree programme in the Health Sciences (Brown, 1989).

A multidisciplinary Health Sciences degree was conceptualized because at the time, the health service in Jamaica was experiencing an acute shortage of health professionals and in most instances, the professionals lacked the necessary skills in management and administration. Additionally, the advances internationally in science and health care had increased the societal and individual expectations for greater and better health care.

The rationale for the development of the Course of Study was explained by Roper & Sangster, (1989) as follows:

- No other Course of Study existed in the region for the upgrading of professionals in their specific areas to the degree level.
- The Course of Study involved the strengthening and ongoing development of a national institution to deliver these advanced courses of study.
- The Course of Study provides for upward mobility and career development of persons in their professional area. These professionals were demoralized and had lost hope of further training outside of going overseas either temporarily or permanently by migration.
- The Course of Study provides for an interdisciplinary team approach to a wide spectrum of health professionals who have previously operated on their own.
- The health services require professionals with management skills to implement health policies and plans for proper delivery of the health services.

The design recognized the existing education and training in the various health disciplines which would comprise the multidisciplinary degree. In so doing, it transferred the diploma credits towards the degree certification, making the Health Sciences degree a post-diploma degree. Figure 1 outlines the Course of Study design for the Multi-disciplinary Bachelor of Health Sciences degree (Roper & Sangster, 1989).

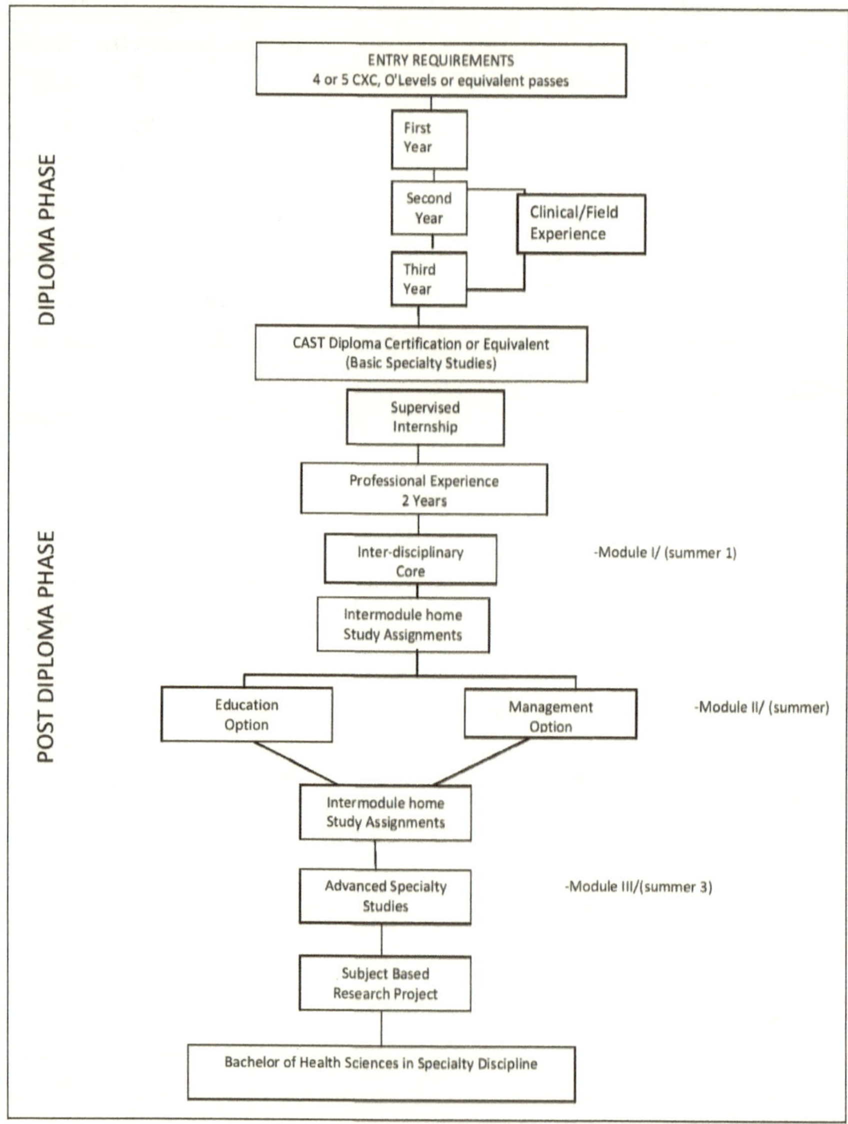

Figure 1: The CAST Multi-disciplinary Bachelor of Health Science Degree Programme

Persons enrolling for the post-diploma degree were expected to successfully complete a course of study in a particular health discipline or specialization leading to the basic proficiency certification. In addition, a minimum of two years post-diploma professional working experience in the discipline in which the student intended to pursue advanced (degree) studies was required.

The Post-diploma phase of the Course of Study consisted of three modules, initially to be delivered over three consecutive summers (see module 1, 2 and 3 below):

- Module 1   Interdisciplinary Core courses
- Module 2   Optional Tracts with studies designed to provide the necessary skills in either management or education (teaching methods)
- Module 3   Advanced Specialty Studies or discipline-specific course of study

In the case of Pharmacy, the aims of the post-diploma phase were to:

a. Educate and train pharmacists to practice outside of the traditional roles and extend their involvement to areas of Clinical Pharmacy, Drug Research and Development and Drug Analysis.
b. Provide education and training which would enable students to develop the skills and confidence to function as effective educators and pharmacy managers.

The curriculum structure for the Pharmacy specialization included the following:

Course	Total Hours	Credits
Biopharmaceutics/Pharmacokinetics	30	2
Drug Information and Drug Literature Evaluation	15	1
Pathology	30	2
Pharmaceutical Technology/ Industrial Pharmacy	60	4

Pharmacology	45	3
Professional Practice	30	2
Research Project	45	3
Therapeutics	45	3
Professional Electives (Choice of 1 out of 3)	30	2
Clinical Clerkship	100	3
Total	**430**	**25**

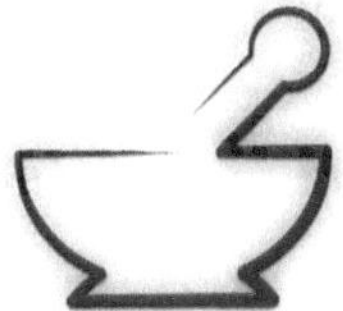

4.

Early Clinical Pharmacy Initiatives

CLINICAL TRAINING FOR PHARMACISTS

Post graduate Training Programme in Clinical Pharmacy

A postgraduate training programme in clinical pharmacy was offered for graduates of the CAST Diploma in Pharmacy in 1974. The programme was introduced because graduates prior to that time had no opportunity to be exposed to the clinical application of pharmacy, that is, direct interaction with physicians, nurses and patients. Because the existing 6-month internship was not providing the clinical experience, the MOH and Environmental Control agreed to supplement the customary training with a tutorship in Clinical Pharmacy.

Whereas, the clinical pharmacy training was a widely accepted part of pharmacy education and practice in North America, it was not being offered in the Caribbean. It was decided that teaching an introductory course in Clinical Pharmacy could be appropriately introduced into the Internship component to provide a goal-oriented learning experience. The Clinical Pharmacy course involved 160 hours of tutorship at the KPH or UHWI through their respective departments of pharmacy. According to the authors, Strein and Mallman (1975), the objective was to provide the maximum exposure possible to patients utilizing drugs, to those health professionals and departments directly involved with the use of drugs, and to the elements of the role of pharmacy in total patient care.

The training was conducted by George W. Strein Jr. and Jack C. Mallman, pharmacists of Project HOPE in Jamaica, under the direction of the MOH. It was specifically designed for the pharmacy class of 1974, a total of thirty students. The graduates received one month of valuable instruction and exposure to clinical pharmacy with emphasis on total patient care and the improvement of pharmaceutical services within the hospital setting. The programme was conducted simultaneously at both hospitals, with one HOPE pharmacist supervising at each institution. The programme was part-funded by the ALCOA Foundation, Jamaica.

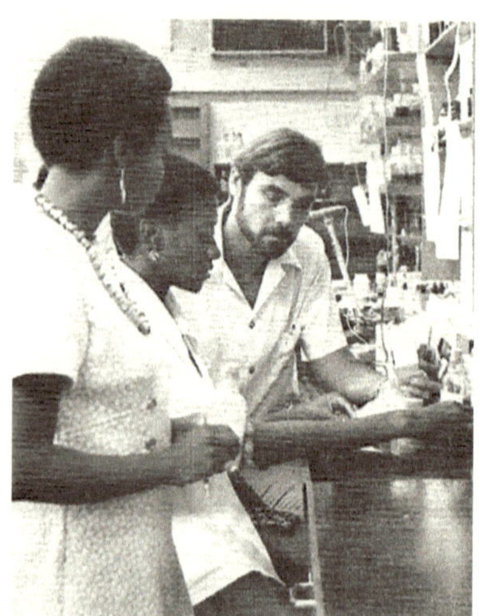

Figure 1. George W. Strein

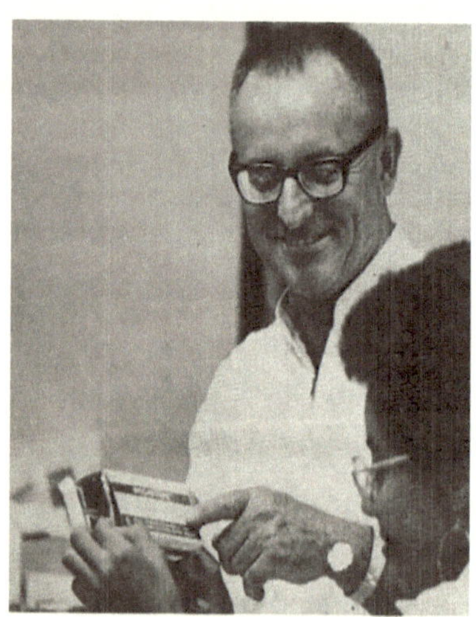

Figure 2. Jack C. Mallman

Clinical Training as part of Internship Programme

In November 1990, a contract was entered into in Kingston, Jamaica between the Ministry of Health, referred to as the "Contracting Agency" and Eugenie Brown (now Eugenie Brown-Myrie), Clinical Pharmacist, the Contractor. The Statement of Services detailed the terms of reference of the agreement as set out below: (see full contract in Appendix 2 a–c)

Statement of Services

The Clinical component of the Pharmacy Internship Programme serves to expose pharmacy students on their practical experience to some of the clinical operations in a large hospital. The programme will be conducted on a rotation basis.

Each rotation will last for approximately six (6) weeks. The Contractor shall:

1. Conduct at least two (2) rotations for each class of interns
2. Make independent rounds to familiarize herself with the cases on the wards as preparation for participating on rounds and to be able to verify information presented by students
3. Conduct approximately (two or) three ward rounds per week for interns at the same time as Medical Rounds and in conjunction with the Medical Team;(depending on hospital used and duration of Medical Rounds)
4. Conduct lectures and group discussions twice weekly
5. Supervise Case Presentations to alternate with lecture sessions
6. Conduct at least one seminar per rotation
7. Administer three (3) quizzes per rotation and a final examination
8. Submit to the Director of the Pharmaceutical Division, Ministry of Health, a general report at the end of each rotation and relevant progress reports on each intern.

5.

The UTech, Jamaica Era: Undergraduate Offerings

CAST AWARDED UNIVERSITY STATUS

The College of Arts, Science & Technology was formally accorded University status on September 1, 1995 as the University of Technology, Jamaica. The University of Technology, Jamaica Act 27-1999, which made permanent provisions for the establishment of the University of Technology, Jamaica was approved by Parliament on June 8, 1999 and signed into law by the Governor General on June 19, 1999 (UTech, Jamaica Summary of Programmes, 2012–13).

EVOLUTION TO THE BACHELOR OF PHARMACY

Prior to the availability of a Bachelor of Pharmacy Course of Study in Jamaica, several pharmacist-graduates of CAST went to Universities in the United Kingdom through the instrumentality of the Pharmaceutical Services Division, Ministry of Health to upgrade to a Bachelors' degree status. Among these early pioneers were Lester Woolery, Granville Forbes, Hermine Metcalfe and Grace Allen-Young. Graduates from the CAST-

Howard collaborations were also pace-setters in this journey towards the Bachelor of Pharmacy among Jamaican pharmacists.

Others, through their own instrumentality pursued doctoral studies overseas. Some of these individuals returned to Jamaica and made significant contribution to the advancement of the profession in the 1970s–1990s. Hugh Lunan and Yvonne Crichton were among the Doctoral graduates who returned to share their knowledge.

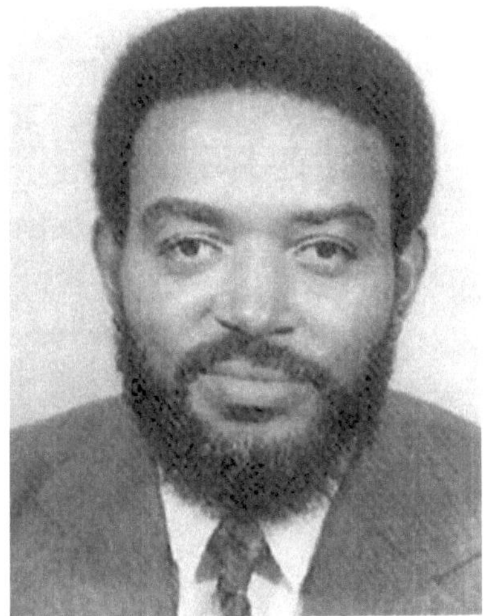

Figure 3. Hugh Noris Lunan

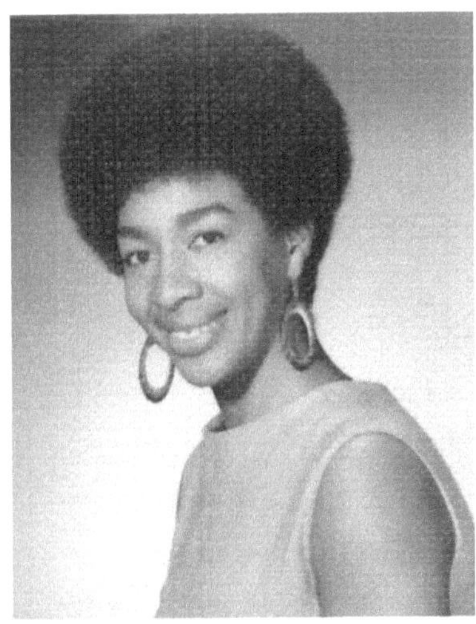

Figure 4. Yvonne Crichton

The offering of a degree was considered because for more than thirty (30) years the University of Technology, Jamaica (formerly C.A.S.T.) produced Diploma graduates in Pharmacy for Jamaica and many other Caribbean countries. These graduates provided quality pharmaceutical and other health care-related services in their respective countries.

However, despite this fruitful and long tradition, the Diploma in Pharmacy Course of Study at the University of Technology, Jamaica, formerly, C.A.S.T., was no longer acceptable in the international arena. All the indicators suggested that the education and training needed to mature into a degree level Course of Study. The rationale for this much needed progression was supported from several perspectives:

Firstly, there was need for upgrading in academic and practical pharmacy training to keep pace with the many changes in pharmacy practice, internationally and in how health care was currently being delivered. Therefore, the necessity arose for pharmacists to be made aware of current knowledge and trends to become competent professionals who would function as drug specialists and integral members of the health care team.

The development of a degree Course of Study was also necessary to comply with international and local professional standards. For example, the Caribbean Association of Pharmacists had stipulated that by the year 2000, the minimum entry requirement to the profession would be a B. Pharm. Degree. For the Caribbean region, the planned inauguration of the Caribbean Pharmacy Examination Board (CARIPEB) would also require candidates with a B. Pharm. or equivalent qualification to write the examination.

Here in Jamaica, the Pharmacy Council through the Ministry of Health considered making the Bachelor of Pharmacy the minimum entry qualification for pharmacist licensure. Finally, upgrading of academic qualifications was a requirement for international academic recognition. This would ensure recognition at international professional fora as well as provide opportunities locally and abroad for further education and or employment (Course Rationale, 1994).

As stated earlier, in 1995, the College of Arts Science and Technology transitioned to The University of Technology, Jamaica (UTech, Jamaica). At that time the Bachelor of Health Sciences (Pharmacy) offering, was discontinued after two cycles producing two batches of graduates. This was replaced by the Post Diploma Summer modular delivery of the Bachelor of Pharmacy.

The Bachelor of Pharmacy Degree abbreviated as "B. Pharm." was introduced at the UTech, Jamaica first in 1995 as a Post-Diploma offering, building on the three-year Diploma certification offered by the CAST training (Appendix 3 – Course of Study structure of last Diploma curriculum). In 1996, one year after CAST became a university, the institution introduced the 4-year, full-time Bachelor of Pharmacy (B. Pharm.) degree.

B.Pharm. Course of Study Goals

Two general Course of Study goals which guided the academic delivery were: (1) to educate and equip persons to provide an acceptable level of pharmacy practice in an evolving patient care environment and (2) to provide a sound base for graduates to pursue further studies in technical, professional or managerial disciplines.

B.Pharm. Course of Study Objectives

The specific objectives were to provide the theoretical knowledge and help develop the clinical skills necessary for professional practice, develop problem solving skills, train pharmacy practitioners to function efficiently in pharmacy and pharmaceutical settings of industrial, hospital and community practice. Additionally, they were to provide graduates with basic training in pharmacy administration and managerial capacity and foster an environment that will encourage graduates to pursue research or further studies in pharmacy and related areas.

POST-DIPLOMA COURSE OFFERINGS

Face-to-Face Offering

The Post-Diploma Degree was introduced in 1995 to provide opportunities for persons who had been trained to the Diploma level to be upgraded to the degree level. Because the course was for practicing pharmacists, delivery modalities were identified so that there would not be disruption of service in organizations. Jamaican pharmacists at home as well as those who resided outside of Jamaica grasped the opportunity. Other Caribbean nationals also seized the opportunity. The following delivery modalities were provided:

- 1-year full time
- 3 summers (Modular)

A 5-week clinical rotation at the end of the didactic training was required for both modalities.

The Post-Diploma Course of Study recognised the previous credits earned from the University's Pharmacy Diploma or equivalent courses of study from recognised institutions. The Diploma component consisted of a minimum of 90 credits (each credit is equivalent to 15 contact hours or 30–45 laboratory hours). It was conducted either on a summer modular basis over three consecutive summers, with each module being of 12 weeks' duration or over three academic sessions, two semesters and a summer session (one-year full-time). In addition to the didactic aspect, students were required to complete an independent research project and a 5-week clinical rotation. Applicants to the Course of Study were required to complete a minimum of two years of post-diploma work experience. In addition, the applicant was required to successfully pass a qualifying exam and/or interview or evaluation of other qualifications. It was projected that the delivery of the Post-Diploma Course of Studyy would continue based on demand. The face-to-face option was phased out and replaced by a fully online offering in academic year 2013–14. (See Appendix 4 for the Post-Diploma Curriculum).

The Post-Diploma face-to-face underwent several reviews with minor adjustments to the curriculum during the eighteen years of its face-to-face delivery. When the enrolment into the course became too small for the offering to be economically viable, the Course of Study was converted to on-line delivery.

Online Offering

In the academic year 2013–14, the Post-Diploma on-line, 2-year full time course ("the first online degree in the Caribbean") was introduced. Students from St Lucia, Barbados, Anguilla, Grenada, Antigua & Barbuda and Jamaica enrolled in the first cohort of the Course of Study.

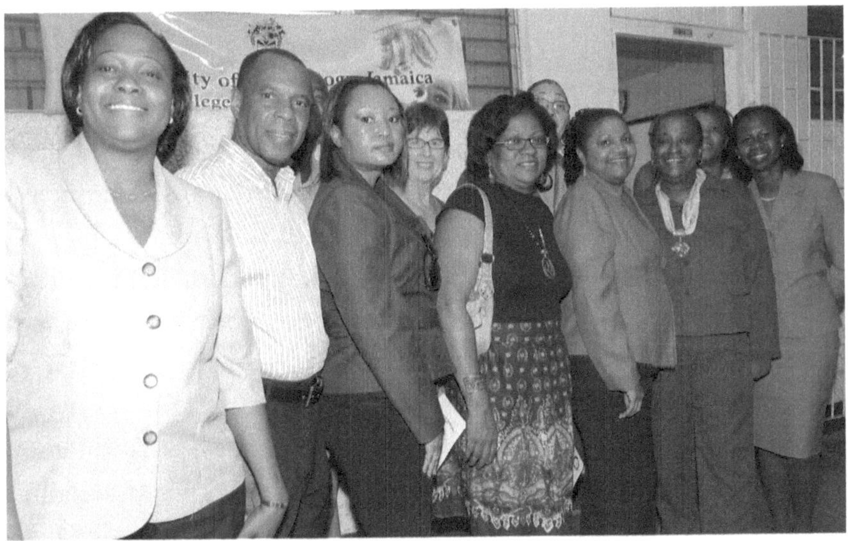

Figure 5. UTech, Jamaica staff of Online Programme and Caribbean Partners
Left to right: (Front Row): Novlette Mattis-Robinson (Programme Director,
UTech, Jamaica), Christine Fray-Aiken (UTech, Jamaica), Evelyn Davis (Gre-
nada), Juliette Gordon (Lecturer, UTech, Jamaica), Dean Ellen Campbell-
Grizzle (UTech, Jamaica), Janet Campbell-Shelly (Vice Dean, UTech, Jamaica).
Back Row: Francis Burnett (St Lucia) Lisa Proverbs (Barbados), Thelma Nelson,
(Chair, Pharmacy Council of Jamaica), Bartley Bryan (Dr Jeanette M. Bartley
Bryan, Ass.VP, Office of Distant Learning, UTech, Jamaica). *Third Row*: Carlyon
Russell, LTSU, UTech, Jamaica)

Associate Professor Ellen Campbell-Grizzle, Dean of the College of
Health Sciences remarked that the online Course of Study was a convenient
vehicle to support the CARICOM harmonization agreement. This
agreement stated that all pharmacists should have a Bachelor of Pharmacy
degree to work in CARICOM states. She further remarked that the online
pharmacy degree ensured that UTech, Jamaica could offer this option
to governments who do not wish to release their valued pharmacists for
two-year periods to engage in the upgrading process. Importantly, the
students apply directly to UTech, Jamaica, and would not be part of any
franchise agreement (*The Observer*, Thursday, May 30, 2013).

The UTech, Jamaica Pharmacy online degree was supported by a

European Union Grant of 100,000 Euros that was awarded to UTech, Jamaica, for the start-up training of the pharmacists in St Lucia in the first round. The project was intended to pay for full tuition fees for students, their per diem during clinical clerkship, content writing and capacity building for pharmacy preceptors in St Lucia. Contributors to the project development were Associate Professor, Dean Ellen Campbell-Grizzle, Dr Sean Moncrieffe and the Ministry of Health in St Lucia. The College of Health Sciences, at UTech, Jamaica negotiated with other Eastern Caribbean States for similar support for their pharmacists. The UTech, Jamaica School of Pharmacy, viewed as the best in the Caribbean, was at the time headed by Dr Sean Moncrieffe. Mrs Novlette Mattis-Robinson was the Programme Director responsible for the first offering of the online degree programme at the time.

Of the 40 students who enrolled, only 28 continued into the second academic year (AY 2014–2015). In academic year 2014/15, a second cohort was accepted for the online delivery. This time 28 students were offered acceptance places. However, attrition resulted in only nine of the 28 students continuing in the Course of Study. Reasons cited for the attrition included: financial constraints, time management issues, family commitments, lack of familiarity with use of technology and the online delivery modality. Some measures employed by the School of Pharmacy to address the challenges faced by the students included the provision of a 3-year completion option, over nine semesters, recruitment and increased involvement and interface of an Online Instructional Liaison Officer, increased involvement of the Office of Distance Learning, Programme Director and Site Coordinators.

Having completed the didactic component of the Course of Study, the first group of students to commence the Clinical component met at the UTech, Jamaica, School of Pharmacy for the Clinical Orientation exercise in June 2015.

Supervision for the Clinical Rotation was provided by Dr Juliette Gordon, Clerkship Coordinator and Lecturer. The rotation sites were Kingston Public Hospital, University Hospital of the West Indies and

Cornwall Regional Hospital. During the clinical clerkship period, the students were exposed to all specializations within the hospital system, participated in ward rounds and were tutored by the pharmacists in those settings. Another batch of students from the first cohort arrived in Jamaica in September 2015 for clinical clerkship. These included pharmacists from Barbados, Anguilla, Belize and Grenada. In November 2015, fifteen students graduated from the first cohort.

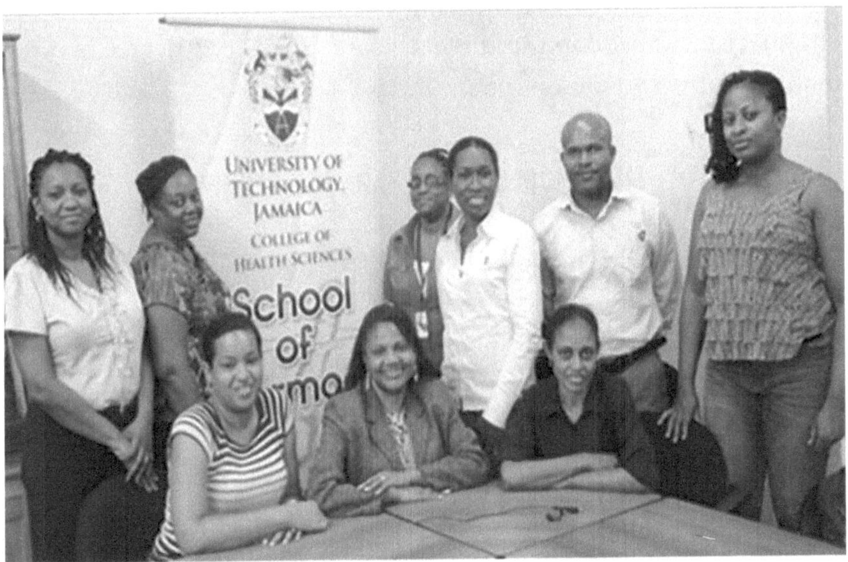

Figure 6. First Cohort of Online Post-Diploma Students
Left to right: (Standing): Laurencia Jean (St Lucia), Nadine Walker, Sophia Morgan, Simone Pinkney, Glenford Ferril, Ebanga Obenson (Jamaica). *Sitting from left:* Carolyn Roman-Dawson, Dr Juliette Gordon (Clerkship Coordinator/Lecturer), Lisa Cheong (St Lucia) at a special meeting held at the College of Health Sciences, Papine campus on Tuesday, June 2, 2015.

In addressing the students, Associate Professor, Ellen Campbell-Grizzle, Dean of the College of Health Sciences on June 2, 2015 said that the School of Pharmacy was engaged in a major pharmacy transformation and regional harmonization. She noted with pleasure that the students would be among the first cohort who would graduate in November 2015.

This online course of study was in keeping with the quest for Regional harmonization and free movement of pharmacy professionals. Under the Curacoa Accord (2001), pharmacists in the Caribbean Association of Pharmacists (CAP) agreed to this minimum qualification for professional practice. This decision was conveyed to CARICOM. Thus, Caribbean pharmacists were required to upgrade from Associate Degrees or Diplomas to a Bachelor's degree. This online Course of Study was a convenient vehicle to support the CARICOM harmonization agreement that required all pharmacists to have a minimum Bachelor of Pharmacy degree in order to work in different nation states.

FOUR-YEAR FULL TIME BACHELOR OF PHARMACY DEGREE

The Bachelor of Pharmacy (B.Pharm.) Course of Study aims to train individuals to become competent and compassionate health care professionals with a commitment to the welfare of patients. The course of study emphasizes current knowledge and skills to enable graduates to meet the demands of society's health care needs as they relate to pharmacy practice. It also provides a sound foundation for graduates to pursue further education and professional qualifications.

Persons wishing to enroll in the Course of Study must satisfy the following requirements:

1. meet matriculation requirements, which is a minimum of five (5) subjects at CXC (CSEC) General Proficiency Grades I, II and III or GCE 'O' Levels A, B or C in Mathematics. English, Chemistry, Biology and one other science-related subject, preferably Physics. In addition, the candidate should obtain two (2) GCE 'A' Levels grades A, to E or CAPE (Units I & II) grades I to V in Chemistry (compulsory), Biology, Zoology, Mathematics or Physics. Passes for the above subjects should be obtained in not more than two sittings

2. applicants are required to attend and be successful at a selection interview

3.   meet the financial requirement for the Course of Study (self-financing, student loan, scholarships, or combination)

4.   be successful at the Psychometric Evaluation (introduced in AY 2009–10)

EXPERIENTIAL COMPONENT OF THE BACHELOR OF PHARMACY COURSE OF STUDY

Clinic Duty

Clinic duty (experience in the CAST/UTech Pharmacy) was introduced in the 3rd year of the Pharmacy Curriculum in 1974. The History of the CAST/UTech Pharmacy reveals that the original dispensary or shop was first licensed by the Drugs and Poisons Board on January 21, 1974. Clinic Duty exposes students to the inner workings of a community pharmacy and includes dispensing of medications, patient counseling and pharmacy inventory. Students attend scheduled one-hour sessions in the UTech Pharmacy, where they interact with patients, engage in the dispensing functions and complete assigned exercises which enhance their learning. The experiential component in the Pharmacy has undergone many revisions over the years as student numbers increased or the programme offering was upgraded. The Clinic Duty is now a well-structured unit attached to the Dispensing II Module, and it also contributes to the overall credit weighting of the Course of Study.

Clerkship/Externships

The pharmacy clerkship/externship rotations are the final component of the professional practice curriculum of the Bachelor of Pharmacy Course of Study. This experiential training provides opportunities for the students to apply their academic knowledge and their problem solving and decision-making skills. The practical experience acquaints the student with the roles of pharmacists in the tertiary care hospital and in community practice. Through this experience the pharmacy student develops skills to function as part of the health care team, through their interactions with the patients and other health care professionals.

Practice experience coordinated by the University of Technology, Jamaica, allows students to apply their knowledge, skills and attitudes during pharmacy practice. During the Clerkship and Externship components of the Course of Study, students get hands-on experience relating to various aspects of pharmacy practice and management. The three main areas of the Clerkship/Externship experiential learning include the Community Externship, Hospital Externship and Clinical Clerkship.

The Clerkship/Externship training is divided into 3 five-week rotations, requiring a minimum of 40 hours per week. The student is required to visit the School of Pharmacy during weeks 2, 3 and 5 for Seminars, Discussions and Evaluation meetings.

Community Externship

This is a practical experience coordinated by the University but is conducted in community pharmacies. Academic credits are awarded for the practical experience.

Preceptors are selected for the supervision of students during their assignment at the pharmacies. This rotation provides the environment for students to demonstrate competences in communicating with patients and other health professions, identifying and resolving drug related problems, selecting and making recommendations for non-prescription medications and providing appropriate patient education and counselling.

Hospital Externship

Students complete a five-week rotation while assigned to a Hospital Pharmacy. During the rotation, competence is assessed in the areas of communication skills, drug information, drug therapy monitoring, conducting medication histories and patient counseling. The goal is to work with other health care professionals in the hospital to optimise patient care.

Clinical Clerkship

The clinical rotation for Bachelor of Pharmacy students is designed to facilitate development of competences in the provision of clinical and pharmaceutical services. It provides an opportunity for the application of knowledge gained in therapeutics, pharmacokinetics, drug information retrieval and evaluation and verbal and written communication in a patient-care (clinical) setting. The student will practice patient monitoring and deliver case presentations as they relate to the medical conditions encountered on the rotation.

On successful completion of the four-year full-time Bachelor of Pharmacy Course of Study, graduates are awarded the UTech, Jamaica Bachelor of Pharmacy degree. This achievement qualifies the graduate to enroll in the Internship (vocational training) programme administered by the Pharmacy Council of Jamaica. At the end of the Internship Training, the Pharmacy Intern becomes eligible for registration to practice Pharmacy in Jamaica. Two graduates of the first cohort of the four-year full-time degree programme shared their reflections on different aspects of the education and training obtained during their Course of Study (See Appendix 5)

The Pharmacy Internship

Upon graduation with a B. Pharm degree, graduates must complete one (1) year internship (vocational training) as a prerequisite for the issuance of a license and registration to practice as a Pharmacist in Jamaica as stipulated under the Pharmacy Act of 1966. Details of the internship programme will be covered in Chapter 7.

Community Experience Required by the Pharmacy Council of Jamaica

In 1995, the Pharmacy Council introduced a requirement for all persons requiring registration to complete 500 hours of Community hours. These

500 hours must be completed by the end of internship. Currently, 400 of those hours must be completed by the end of year 4 of the Pharmacy Course of Study and the remaining 100 hours during the internship period. Students receive credit for 200 hours towards the Community Externship from their UTech, Jamaica Community Externship rotation completed in year four of the 4-year full-time B.Pharm Course of Study. Preceptors are approved by Pharmacy Council of Jamaica (PCJ) for the Community Externship Course of Study.

UTECH, JAMAICA-COLLEGE OF THE BAHAMAS (COB) FRANCHISE

In 2008, the University of Technology, Jamaica and the College of the Bahamas signed an agreement to facilitate the delivery of the Bachelor of Pharmacy degree Course of Study in the Commonwealth of the Bahamas (see Appendix 6, UTech-COB Franchise Agreement, June 2008). In the initial stage, the agreement was for the students to complete the first two years of the Course of Study in the Bahamas and the latter two at the Kingston campus of the University of Technology, Jamaica. The agreement sought to train approximately twenty-five students in each cohort. However, the numbers did not materialize. There were 18 enrollees in the first cohort, 14 became graduates. Only eight students enrolled in the second cohort. Two cohorts completed the Course of Study under this arrangement, with a total of twenty-one graduating with the Bachelor of Pharmacy degree.

The initial agreement was revised in academic year 2012/13 to allow for the full delivery of the Course of Study at the College of the Bahamas. At the time of writing, one cohort of students had completed the Course of Study under the revised agreement and another class was progressing through the fourth year of study.

BSC IN PHARMACEUTICAL TECHNOLOGY

The BSc in Pharmaceutical Technology was introduced in academic year 2014–15. The course seeks to provide individuals with the requisite skills for employment in pharmaceutical manufacturing, production, development as well as operations and analysis sectors. Graduates can find employment in the local, regional and international pharmaceutical industry. Spanish has been included in the course so that graduates will be marketable in both English and Spanish speaking regions.

The new training in Pharmaceutical Technology is in keeping with UTech, Jamaica's mandate to continuously expand its academic offerings to meet current local, regional and global labour market needs for development.

The four-year BSc in Pharmaceutical Technology Course of Study was the first for any training institution in the English-speaking Caribbean. It provides students with broad-based training skills that are required to work in the pharmaceutical industry with particular emphasis on drug manufacturing, pharmaceutical production and development. The introduction of this prestigious degree offering added a new dimension to the enviable reputation for excellence in pharmacy education that the University has enjoyed over its half a century of Course of Study offerings (See Appendix 7 – Course Brochure).

The official launch of the Course of Study took place on February 26, 2015 at a ceremony held at the Petroleum Corporation of Jamaica (PCJ) auditorium in Kingston. The Programme Director, Dr Marcia Williams in providing an overview of the course stated that during years 3 and 4 of the Course of Study, students would spend five weeks in the field and in the last Semester of the fourth-year students would be required to complete an externship in a manufacturing plant. She highlighted that an important feature of the programme was a four-level Spanish course, which would enable graduates to communicate more effectively internationally, particularly, with neighbours in Latin America where the pharmaceutical industry was growing.

Dean Ellen Campbell-Grizzle in her comments at the launch predicted that the historic significance of the new Course of Study is that it would produce pharmaceutical science graduates who would "become important high-level knowledge workers in what is to become a period of great restoration in the pharmaceutical, nutraceutical and cosmoceutical manufacturing industry in Jamaica". She added that the course of study was particularly relevant, considering current demand for knowledge-based competency in the exploration of indigenous plants such as cannabis for research and application for medicinal, pharmaceutical and industrial uses.

PROGRAMME ACCREDITATION

Accreditation is a method of External Quality Assurance (EQA). This is the method of EQA utilized by the University Council of Jamaica (UCJ). The UCJ which was established by the University Council of Jamaica Act, 1987 is the National Quality Assurance Agency for tertiary education in Jamaica.

The process of accreditation is intended to strengthen and sustain the quality of tertiary education so that it is worthy of public confidence. Accreditation is the status granted to programmes or institutions by Accreditation bodies when established standards for educational quality are met or exceeded. Self-study and peer review processes must be carried out (UCJ, 2017).

The University of Technology, Jamaica (UTech, Jamaica) is committed to excellence in all aspects of its course offerings. By submitting its courses of study to accrediting bodies for review and accreditation, the University ensures that its courses of study are of the highest quality and meet international standards (Ellis, 2009). The University of Technology, Jamaica is guided by the Academic Quality Audit Policy (2011). The Pharmacy course of study undergoes regular quality audits to ensure on-going quality of the course and modules offered to students. The process aims not only to ensure quality, but to assist with programme accreditation, strengthen the institution in its move towards institutional accreditation, as well as, improve the data collection capabilities of the School of Pharmacy (Moncrieffe, 2014, memo to Pharmacy staff).

The Purpose/Importance of Accreditation (UCJ, 2017) is to assure

Educational Quality and Institutional Integrity. In fulfilling its purposes, accreditation provides services to its general constituencies: institutions, their students, the public and other stakeholders

UTECH, JAMAICA PHARMACY PROGRAMME ACCREDITATION

The Bachelor of Pharmacy Course of Study received its first UCJ accreditation on May 1, 2000. The Commonwealth Pharmacists Association highlighted the Pharmacy Programme Accreditation in its *CPA Newsletter* in May 2001. (see Appendix 8)

Each accreditation cycle lasted for 4 or 5 years. Renewals were received from the UCJ on May 10, 2004, and again in 2010 (granted late). The submission for the third re-accreditation (Fourth Accreditation Certificate was sent to the UCJ in 2013. The third accreditation was granted for a five year period; an extension from the previous four year accreditation periods. The *Jamaica Gleaner* recognized these accreditations by reporting that the renewal of accreditations for each cycle was received from the UCJ (*Jamaica Gleaner*, 2017).

TYPES OF ACCREDITATION

Programme Accreditation is the evaluation of the quality of specific programmes offered by an institution against established criteria.

Institutional Accreditation is a comprehensive evaluation of an institution and its academic as well as administrative effectiveness. There is focus on the institution's Internal Quality Assurance Systems.

Professional Accreditation is the public recognition accorded to a professional program that meets established professional qualifications and educational standards through initial and periodic evaluation. These Accreditation Standards reflect those professional and educational attributes identified by the Council as essential for programs intending to develop practicing clinical patient focused pharmacists (Canadian Council for Accreditation of Pharmacy Programs, 2014).

In the United States of America, the Accreditation Council for Pharmacy Education (ACPE) is the public body responsible for the professional accreditation. It recognises that the professional degree program leading to the Doctor of Pharmacy degree is judged to meet established qualifications and education standards through initial and subsequent periodic evaluations. ACPE is recognized by the US Department of Education (USDE) for the accreditation and pre-accreditation, within the United States, of professional degree programs in pharmacy leading to the degree of Doctor of Pharmacy (https://www.acpe-accredit.org/pharmd-program-accreditation/).

Institutional Accreditation Status

The University of Technology, Jamaica, was granted Institutional Accreditation on December 13, 2018, effective from February 20, 2018 to February 19, 2025. Having obtained Institutional Accreditation, it means that all degree programmes offered by the university are recognised by the UCJ, local and international stakeholders, as meeting minimum acceptable standards.

The University of the West Indies currently has Institutional Accreditation from the UCJ. As such, its Pharmacy programme will be automatically accredited. Information in the institution's Pharmacy Curriculum, reveals that it intends to apply for Regional Accreditation from the Caribbean Accreditation Agency for Medicine and other Health Professionals (CAAM-HP) in the near future.

Professional Accreditation Status

Investigations are ongoing that will lead to Professional Accreditation of the Pharmacy Course of Study in the shortest possible time.

6.

Institutionalization:
Graduate Offerings and Professional Degrees

UTECH, JAMAICA GRADUATE OFFERINGS

Master/Doctor of Philosophy Degrees in Pharmaceutics/ Pharmaceutical Technology

The MPhil Pharmaceutics/Pharmaceutical Technology and PhD Pharmaceutics/Pharmaceutical Technology are both offered with full-time or part-time options. This degree is the first of its kind in the Caribbean. Graduates trained in pharmaceutical dosage forms, process research and development as well as manufacturing and control are expected to contribute significantly to pharmaceutical research and development in Jamaica and the Caribbean.

The Masters Course of Study has two options:

MPhil in Pharmaceutics

The entry requirement for the M Phil in Pharmaceutics is the Bachelor's degree in Pharmacy (UTech, Jamaica, or any other institution recognized by the Academic Board). The Pharmaceutics option comprises 42 academic credits, twenty of which are accounted for as taught modules and twenty-two towards the Research.

MPhil in Pharmaceutical Technology

Persons wishing to pursue the Pharmaceutical Technology track must hold a Bachelor of Pharmacy or B.Sc. in Applied Chemistry, Industrial or Analytical Chemistry, Biochemistry or related area from UTech, Jamaica or any other institution approved by the Academic Board.

The Doctor of Philosophy (PhD) in Pharmaceutics

Persons wishing to enroll in the PhD Course of Study should hold an M Phil in Pharmaceutics/ Pharmaceutical Technology or a taught Master's degree in Pharmacy with a strong research component.

By 2016, four cohorts of graduates from the M Phil in Pharmaceutics were produced and in that same year the first candidate enrolled for the Doctor of Philosophy Course of Study.

Post Baccalaureate Doctor of Pharmacy (PharmD)

Since the early eighties, the practice of pharmacy has changed from a primarily distribution role to one which has placed greater emphasis on the concept of pharmaceutical care. This philosophy of pharmaceutical care has challenged pharmacists with the responsibility for providing drug therapy that achieves defined outcomes and improves a patient's quality of life. There is growing acceptance of this expanded role of the pharmacist, as health care providers realize the added value of pharmacists' input into therapeutic decision-making processes. There is increasing evidence that the pharmacists' intervention can result in cost reduction through prevention of drug-related problems, prescribing or administration errors and patient noncompliance (PharmD Course of Study Curriculum, 2009).

In keeping with the current thrust of the University of Technology, Jamaica (UTech) to strive for excellence and build human capacity, the School of Pharmacy implemented the Post-Baccalaureate Doctor of Pharmacy (PharmD) Course of Study in August 2010. The PharmD course of study at UTech, Jamaica is a post-graduate degree designed for highly motivated pharmacists who hold an accredited Bachelor's degree or equivalent in pharmacy and who desire to advance their educational and professional career. The Course of Study focuses primarily on the therapeutic management of conditions associated with the human biological systems along with elective modules that are unique to the Caribbean region. As a post-baccalaureate degree, the advanced content of the UTech, Jamaica PharmD Course of Study complements practice experience and fosters a higher level of competence and autonomy. The Course of Study includes extensive clinical training that will enable graduates to develop advanced analytical and problem-solving skills and the ability to translate theoretical knowledge into clinical applications (PharmD Curriculum, 2009).

The PharmD Course of Study is intended to equip students to become competent providers of health care and active valued partners in the multi-disciplinary health care team. The graduates will use evidence-based practice to ensure optimal health of the patient and the health-seeking public. The graduates should also be capable of providing leadership in advancing pharmacy practice, research and health policies. The course is delivered in a blended, flexible student-centred learning format within a collaborative learning environment.

The UTech, Jamaica Doctor of Pharmacy degree is offered on a part-time basis, over three calendar years. It comprises nine academic sessions and a total of 78 credits. Seven of the nine semesters/academic sessions cover didactic component of the course; the remaining two semesters focus on the Clinical Rotation Specialties. The didactic component of the course is delivered using a blended modality (face to face and online). Clinical specialties include: Internal Medicine, Paediatrics, Cardiology, Infectious

Diseases, Psychiatry and Trauma Care. Candidates in the Course of Study are also required to complete a Longitudinal Research Project.

Graduates of the PharmD degree are referred to as Clinical Pharmacists. They are qualified to work as clinical specialists, educators and researchers.

Persons desiring to pursue the UTech, Jamaica Post Baccalaureate Doctor of Pharmacy Programme should be registered practicing pharmacists with a Bachelor of Pharmacy (B. Pharm.) or equivalent from an accredited institution. The applicants should have a minimum of a Second Class Honours degree. Applicants with a Pass degree would be required to complete qualifying modules (as determined by the University). Applicants should have at least one year's experience as a practicing pharmacist.

UWI, MONA ENTRY LEVEL DOCTOR OF PHARMACY DEGREE

The PharmD Programme offered by the University of the West Indies (UWI) is a five-calendar year, full-time face to face programme, delivered over fourteen semesters. The pre-clinical (mainly didactic) component of the programme is designed to be completed during the first three years while the fourth and fifth years (clinical component) are primarily devoted to experiential education, where students obtain extensive hands-on clinical experiences in a variety of pharmacy practice settings (UWI Pharmacy Curriculum, 2016).

The programme is designed to prepare graduates to function efficiently as pharmacists in all pharmaceutical settings, inclusive of manufacturing, hospital, distribution and community pharmacies. In order to fit into these settings, the graduate will demonstrate competence in the core knowledge, skills, and practices necessary to solve therapeutic problems.

Criteria for Admission

Applicants wishing to enroll in the Doctor of Pharmacy Programme offered by the University of the West Indies must fulfill the general university regulations concerning matriculations and, the specific requirements of the Faculty of Medical Sciences. Academic requirements for admission to the PharmD are:

1. CAPE Advanced proficiency examinations/GCE A' Level or their equivalent in three (3) subjects, Biology/Zoology and Chemistry. The third subject can be Physics, Mathematics or any other approved subject. The minimum academic standard for entry is an average of two 3's or one B or two C's at GCE A' Level.
2. UWI preliminary or introductory level courses in the appropriate subjects in the Faculty of Pure and Applied Sciences, Mona or Cave Hill, or Faculty of Medical Sciences, or Faculty of Science and Technology and Agriculture, St Augustine, Trinidad.
3. Programme/Courses considered equivalent at institutions recognised by the University of the West Indies.
4. Applicants holding UWI first degrees in the Natural Sciences with a minimum of Lower Second Class Honours may also be considered.
5. Applicants holding professional degrees in Allied Health Disciplines may also be considered for entry, provided that they have attained minimum average grade of B+ or Grade Point of 3.3 in the appropriate science subjects during their degree programme.
6. Applicants who have earned a BSc in Pharmacy from UWI, St Augustine campus or BPharm degree from UTech, Jamaica.

7.

Role of Regulatory Agencies and Professional Associations

PHARMACY INTERNSHIP

The internship programme (vocational training) was introduced for pharmacists after the transfer of responsibility for the education and training to the College of Arts, Science and Technology in 1962. Initially, the vocational training was for six months (interview with Joan Neill, Feb. 28, 2018) then this period was eventually increased to one year. Stafford Haughton (2018), a graduate of the first batch of Pharmacists trained by CAST shared that the internship was completed at two institutions, three months at the University Hospital of the West Indies and three months at the Kingston Public Hospital. There was a transitioning from six months to eight months and finally to one year. John Hall (2003) corroborated the information about internship as he posited in his book that the first batch of graduating students did their internship at the Kingston Public Hospital and the University Hospital of the West Indies. They were exposed to the latest theoretical and practical applications of pharmacy (Hall, 2003).

The authors believe that the extension of internship to one year may have been influenced by the inclusion of the clinical training component into the internship training. This clinical component was not introduced for persons awarded a Diploma until 1994, as a pilot project through the MOH/Eugenie Brown-Myrie (Eugenie Brown then) Contract. It was formally implemented with the introduction of the Bachelor of Pharmacy degree Course of Study in 1996, followed by the internship of 2001.

The PSJ's secretary's report for the period 1988–89, documented that CAST Pharmacy Interns had expressed dissatisfaction with the lack of an organized and cohesive internship programme. The interns submitted recommendations to the then PSJ President, Grace Allen (who later became Dr Grace Allen-Young). The recommendations were forwarded to the Pharmacy Council and copied to the then Director of Pharmaceutical Services, Mr Lester Woolery.

After several years of conducting an internship programme, a *Manual for Pharmacy Internship* (MFPI) was commissioned by the Pharmacy Council of Jamaica. The first author was Ellen Campbell-Grizzle and the publication was in 1996. The Manual was revised in 2003 and 2018. The pharmacy interns have always played a significant role in the development and reviews of the internship programme (Wallace, 2005).

The internship programme aims to produce professionals well-grounded in professional ethics, who are sensitive to the needs of patients and competent to function in all sectors. The programme should instill in candidates that life-long learning is an integral part of the practice of Pharmacy. Additionally, the internship process seeks to encourage positive attitudes among participants. Under the supervision of preceptors, workplace attitudes and ethics will be inculcated that will ensure that "the patient's interest is held paramount over all considerations" (MFPI, 2018).

The *Manual for Pharmacy Internship* in Jamaica (2018) sets out the requirements for the programme. It states that candidates for internship must have been previously registered with the PCJ as Pharmaceutical Students, attended a training institution approved by the PCJ and possess Pharmacy professional entry level qualifications (BPharm or PharmD). They are also required to apply to and obtain placement at approved

Internship sites. A copy of the letter showing confirmation of placement should be submitted to the PCJ.

Other pre-requisites for the internship include completion of four hundred (400) of the required five hundred (500) hours of community experience, submission of the Appendix E (Internship Enrollment Form) with payment of the relevant fees to the PCJ. They are also required to attend the scheduled Pre-Internship Meeting, Orientation Exercise which is **MANDATORY** and to be present at **ALL** Internship Seminars in any given Internship year.

During the early years of the Internship experience, the training was only in Public Sector institutions. The programme was expanded to include training in Community Pharmacies, Distributive and Manufacturing companies. The Pharmacy Council of Jamaica (PCJ) and the Ministry of Health (MOH), Standards and Regulation Division and private sector entities collaborate to ensure appropriate experiential training is provided. Training sites and trained preceptors are approved by PCJ.

REGISTRATION AS A PHARMACIST

The minimum qualification accepted by the Pharmacy Council of Jamaica for registration of a Pharmacist is the Bachelor of Pharmacy degree. Jamaicans and CARICOM nationals trained at an approved institution, who satisfy the requirements for registration, must submit a portfolio containing, the completed application form, certified copy of degrees, three testimonials and the prescribed fee (non-refundable).

CONTINUING EDUCATION REQUIREMENT

The earliest documented record of the delivery of Continuing Education (CE) within the Pharmaceutical Society of Jamaica (PSJ) appeared in *Caribbean Pharmacy News (CPN) News* Vol 1 #4 August/September, 1999. Dr Lester Woolery, then Managing Director at LASCO Pharmaceutical Division in an interview with the Editor of CPN reported that in 1966, he along with Mr Rushworth Haig ("Jeff") Thompson, Mr Von Gladstone Knight and Mr Vincent ("Vin") A. Bennett, Snr. were involved in the delivery of Continuing Education Seminars within the PSJ. Renowned pharmacists such as Linwood Tice, President of the American Society of Hospital Pharmacists, Clifford Jarrett, Head of Canada's Food and Drug Directorate and T.D. Whittett of Britain were invited to Jamaica as presenters at the Seminar (Woolery, 2008, p. 24).

Miss C. Aleen Gray in her article "The History of Pharmacy in Jamaica," made reference to the 1970's as the period when the Pharmaceutical Society of Jamaica initiated Continuing Education Seminars. She acknowledged the work of Mrs Heather Benjamin Alexis, Dr Yvonne Crichton, Mr Keith Golding, Mrs Hermine Metcalfe, Mr George Corrie, Mr Granville Forbes, Mr Leo Vaughn, Mr Dick Kinkead and Mr Paul Ellis in this initiative (Gray, n.d.).

Mr Leonard ("Leo") R. Vaughn in the article, " Of This and That in the Pharmaceutical Society of Jamaica," (*Pharmacy Newsletter*, September-December 1990) made reference to the "on-going Continual Professional Education Programme" which was sponsored by the PSJ since the 1970s. He cited these seminars as a source of extraordinary benefit and assistance to those pharmacists who would avail themselves of the opportunity to attend and participate meaningfully. He posited that he took advantage of the seminars to keep up to date.

The Ministry of Health's efforts in the Continuing Education programme for pharmacists was documented in a correspondence to Dr Eugenie Brown (now Eugenie Brown-Myrie), Pharmacy Programme Director at CAST, requesting her participation in a Seminar for Pharmacists and Pharmacy Technicians, to be held March 1, 1989. Mr Lester Woolery was Director of Pharmaceutical Services at that time (Correspondence to Brown, 1989).

In July 1994, "Guidance on Continuing Education Participation" was developed by Dr Ellen Campbell-Grizzle in collaboration with Dr Yvonne Crichton and Mrs Heather Alexis-Morrison using principles recommended by the Royal Pharmaceutical Society of Great Britain (Grizzle, 1994).

The introduction to the document outlined that in September 1993, the PSJ, at its Annual General Meeting passed a Resolution, that participation in Continuing Education on an annual basis should be a requirement for retention on the register. The Society's decision was based on the premise that it was in the public's interest for pharmacists to be competent and current. The guidance document made reference to efforts being made by PSJ to improve its fifteen (15) year old Continuing Education Programme. The aim was that it would exceed the expectation of Pharmacists (Grizzle, 1994).

PHACE (Pharmacist Active in Continuing Education) was presented to the Pharmacy Council of Jamaica for consideration with the hope that the Council would issue a full statement of support for the concept and begin the process of amending the Pharmacy Act to ensure that the Council's guidelines, in this regard would be mandatory. The advertisement for the PHACE programme which appeared in the 1994 *Pharmacy Magazine* is shown below.

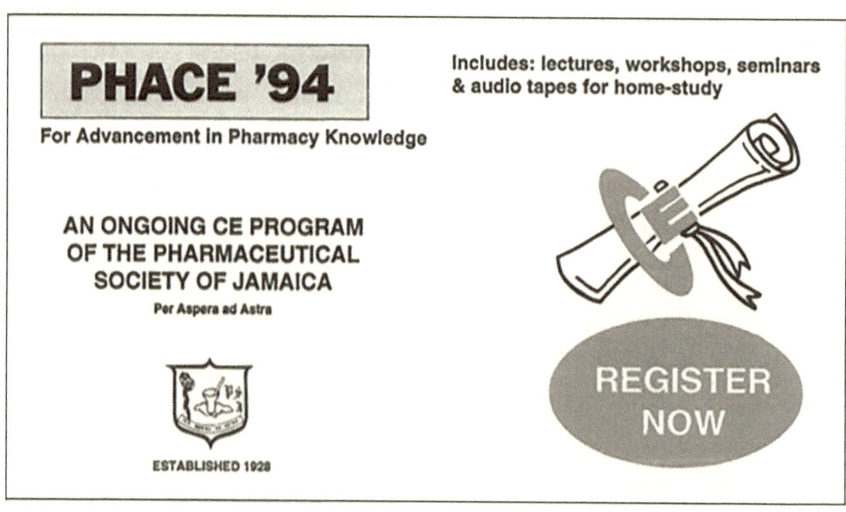

Figure 7. Advertisement for PHACE programme

The Pharmacy (Amendment) Regulations, 2003, which was gazetted Monday, March 31, 2003 established participation in Continuing Education as mandatory for Annual Registration of Pharmacists. The PSJ and APOTEX collaboration pioneered the delivery of continuing education in the early years. The Pharmacy and APOTEX Continuing Education (PACE) Programme booklets (see Representation of Booklet in Appendix 9), along with live CE sessions were hallmarks of that period. In later years, other providers entered the scene/arena. The Pharmacy Council of Jamaica, the Regulatory arm for pharmacists in Jamaica has gone further to introduce a policy, stating that of the twelve (12) CE credits required under Law, all pharmacists are required to obtain a minimum of three (3) credits from seminars provided by the Pharmacy Council of Jamaia (PCJ Update, June 2010).

Some providers of CE Seminars since 2007 include: Pharmaceutical Society of Jamaica (PSJ), Commonwealth Pharmacists Association (CPA), Caribbean Association of Pharmacists (CAP), Caribbean Institute of Pharmacy Practice Policy and Research/University of Technology, Jamaica, Pharmacy Alumni (CIPPPAR/UPA), Cari-Med Ltd and the Pharmacy Council of Jamaica (PCJ).

Various methods have been used to provide continuing education over the years, including live sessions (lectures, workshops, conferences) audiotapes for home study, and prepared booklets. Records reveal that in 2009–2010, Dr Tonoya Toyloy produced a CE booklet on Breast Cancer, which was awarded 1.5 credits (2nd Vice President Andre Morgan's report 2009–10.) With the advancement in technology, pharmacists can also access CE credits through online methods, which include webinars.

The 2009–2010 PSJ Administration expanded the Continuing Education programme to include training of Pharmacists. In its new dispensation, the Committee is called the Continuing Education and Training Committee (CET). The purpose of the committee was to:

- Arrange educational and informative lectures and hold seminars and conferences to enable members to keep a pace of advancements in science and modern pharmacy,
- Facilitate the training of pharmacists in an effort to broaden the

scope of pharmacy and to contribute more holistic care to patients (Bromfield June 19, 2010).

The CET Committee identified and categorized areas in which pharmacists should be trained. The three main categories for training were: Outreach, Therapeutics and Personal Development. In June 2015 the PSJ Conference celebrated 30 years of Quality Continuing Education, that would make 1985 the official start of on-going CE sessions (Pharmaceutical Society of Jamaica, Conference Magazine, June 26–28, 2015).

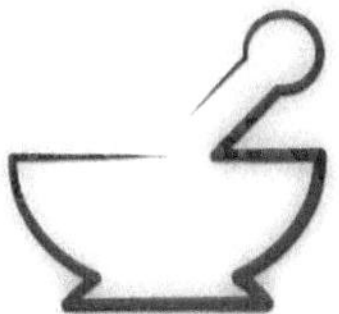

8.

Local, Regional and International Collaborations

Pharmacy education in Jamaica has benefited from the collaboration with academic and training institutions, professional and pharmacy regulatory associations, patient care institutions/facilities, funding agencies, private corporations and pharmacy professionals.

Through the instrumentality of Project HOPE, Washington, DC, there was the development and implementation of a Clinical component in the internship programme for pharmacists trained to the Diploma level. George Strein and Jack Mallman, Project HOPE pharmacists to Jamaica in the 1970s, facilitated the project (Strein and Mallman, 1974). The academic training served as a catalyst for the review and restructuring of the Pharmacy Internship programme in Jamaica.

LOBBY FOR THE BACHELOR OF PHARMACY DEGREE BY PROFESSIONAL AND REGULATORY BODIES

Before the implementation of the Bachelor of Pharmacy degree Course of Study at the University of Technology, Jamaica in 1996, several organizations were instrumental in lobbying for the Bachelor of Pharmacy to be the entry qualification for practicing pharmacists in the Caribbean region. Among the organizations were the Commonwealth Pharmaceutical Association (CPA), Caribbean Association of Pharmacists (CAP), Pharmaceutical Society of Jamaica (PSJ), Pharmacy Council of Jamaica (PCJ) and the Pharmaceutical Services Division of the Ministry of Health (see Appendix 10 – Early Lobbyists for Bachelor of Pharmacy Launch , 1995)

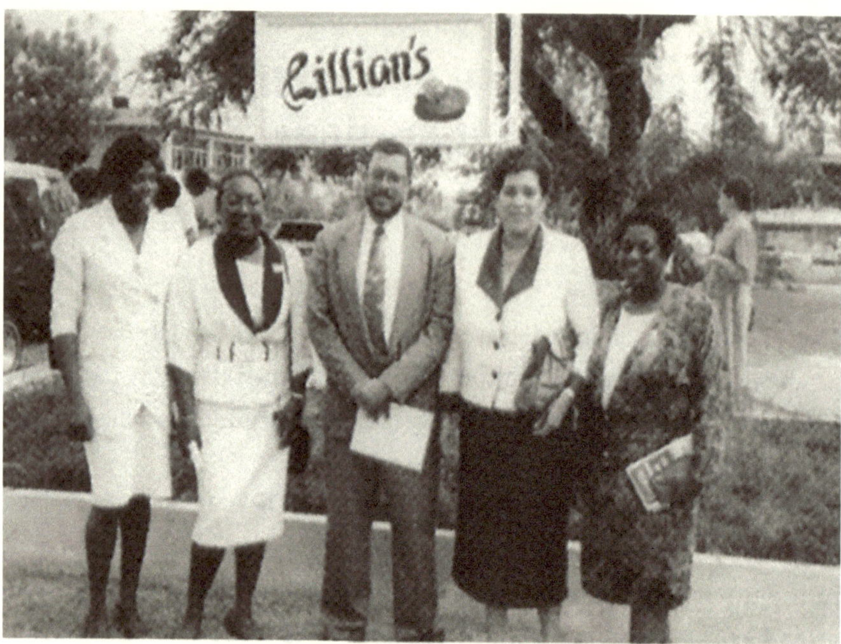

Figure 8. Early Lobbyists for B.Pharm. Launch, 1995
Left to right: Dr Eugenie Brown (Programme Director), Mrs Grace Allen-Young (Director, Pharmaceutical Services Division, Ministry of Health), Dr Peter Phillips (Minister of Health), Miss Thelma Nelson (Chairman, Pharmacy Council of Jamaica) Mrs Ellen Grizzle (President, Pharmaceutical Society of Jamaica).

Dr E. Grace Allen-Young, CPA Council Member reported on the collaboration of significant stakeholders in the implementation of the Bachelor of Pharmacy degree programme in Jamaica. This is the quote from the *CPA Bulletin* in 1995:

In 1991, the CPA Council took the decision that the academic qualification of all pharmacists throughout the commonwealth should be a degree in pharmacy. Armed with this resolution, the Pharmaceutical Services Division of the Ministry of Health, Pharmacy Council of Jamaica, Pharmaceutical Society of Jamaica, the Pharmacy Faculty at the College of Arts, Science and Technology (CAST) and the Pharmacy Advisory Committee succeeded in completing negotiations for the commencement of the Bachelor of Pharmacy Degree at CAST in June 1995.

The Caribbean Association of Pharmacists (CAP) maintained ongoing advocacy for the Bachelor of Pharmacy degree to be the professional entry level qualification for pharmacists. The Curacao Accord records the passing of a Resolution in 2001 at the CAP Conference that year that made this qualification a reality for the Caribbean. Of note, the University of Technology, Jamaica and University of the West Indies, Mount Hope, Trinidad, were already offering the degree in 2000.

FINANCIAL SUPPORT FROM AGENCIES FOR PROGRAMME AND STAFF DEVELOPMENT

The Pan American Health Organization (PAHO) has supported Pharmacy Education in Jamaica through its sponsorship of academic staff to attend the Pan American Conferences on Pharmaceutical Education which are held biennially in Latin American countries and the USA. These conferences have provided a forum for exchange of ideas and the provision of useful training and information for the development and delivery of pharmacy education in Jamaica and the wider Caribbean.

UTech, Jamaica pharmacy students received international exposure though their involvement with the International Pharmacy Student Federation (IPSF), an NGO with the Pan American Health Organization/ World Health Organization (PAHO/WHO). In May 19–23, 2005, the 4th Pan American Regional Symposium was held in Jamaica. This was a first for the Caribbean region. Shameka Jackson, a 4th year UTech, Jamaica Pharmacy student who served on the IPSF Executive was instrumental in getting the Symposium to Jamaica. At that symposium, 58 Jamaican Pharmacy students and 10 pharmacists participated in the event. Through the IPSF connection, Keon Green benefited from a student exchange programme which took her to Sierra Leone in May 2005 (PSJ President's Report, 2005).

The Canadian International Development Agency (CIDA) was instrumental in lending support to Pharmacy Education through Staff (Faculty) development, staff exchange and Continuing Education efforts. Two Faculty members received academic training leading up to the Bachelor of Pharmacy (1991) and MSc Pharmacology (1992), respectively. Professor David Biggs, and Dean of the College of Pharmacy, Professor John Bachynsky, of the University of Alberta, provided support as exchange Faculty, Research Supervisor and Presenters at Continuing Education events during the early 1990s.

In 2003, Mr Sean Moncrieffe, Lecturer at UTech, Jamaica was among the first group of pharmacists trained in distance education techniques at the St. Augustine campus of the UWI, Trinidad. Participants at the training were nominated by CAP and drawn from several academic institutions in the Caribbean. The joint CARICOM/CAP project was funded by CIDA (CPN, 2003).

The contributions of Pharmacists from the United Kingdom, United States of America and Canada must be acknowledged as they supported education efforts through Continuing Education and the establishment of academic programmes which spanned more than a decade and which facilitated upgrading of Jamaican pharmacists to the Bachelor's degree in the United Kingdom. Some of the notable pharmacists were: Mr Linwood Tice from the USA, Clifford Jarrett from Canada and T.D Whittett of the UK (Woolery, 2000).

The Research Development Fund, introduced at the University of Technology, Jamaica, provides an opportunity for staff interested in research to source funding for their scholarly activities. Staff members in the School of Pharmacy who have benefited from this fund have been Drs Sarafadeen Adebayo and Eugenie Brown-Myrie (RDF Final Report, 2005/2006).

PROGRAMME DEVELOPMENT, DELIVERY AND EXPANSION – ACADEMIC INSTITUTIONS

The earliest record of collaboration with an academic institution was the CAST-Howard initiative during the period 1973–1977. This collaboration saw Jamaican pharmacy students in a three year diploma programme travelling to Howard University, Washington, DC, where they had to complete 12 months leading up to the award of a Bachelor of Pharmacy degree. This arrangement lasted for four academic years (Sangster, 2010).

The training of pharmacists in the Bachelor of Health Science (Pharmacy) degree programme benefited from collaboration with University of Texas, Austin. Associate Professor and Head, Clinical Division of the College of Pharmacy at the University of Texas delivered lectures in Clinical Pharmacy and Therapeutics to pharmacy students reading for the Bachelor of Health Science (Pharmacy) degree in 1991. Associate Professor Lynn Crismon also served the College as Consultant, for the Curriculum and Programme Review of the said programme in 1991.

Several projects and grants obtained from Grant Funding Agencies assisted in the development and delivery of Pharmacy education. The Kellogg's Grant, 1986–91 was instrumental in the development and implementation of the Post-Diploma Bachelor of Health Sciences degree programme (Sangster, 2010). The Pharmacy specialization in this Health Science degree was the step towards the introduction of the Bachelor of Pharmacy offering. Miss Janet Campbell (now Janet Campbell-Shelly) was awarded a Fellowship to pursue a Master of Science in Pharmacology at the University of Alberta, 1989–1992. There have been ongoing collaborations with academic institutions over the years, which have benefited staff, graduates and students in the Pharmacy programme. In 2004, the University of Technology, Jamaica and the University of Derby, United Kingdom, entered an agreement for the training of pharmacists to the Master of Science in Clinical Pharmacy. Dr David Gerrett, Head, Pharmacy Academic Practice Unit, University of Derby was the lead person in the discussions leading up to the implementation of the collaboration. The agreement was to establish collaboration between UTech, Jamaica, University Hospital of the West Indies (UHWI) and University of Derby (UOD) to deliver the Master of Science in Clinical Pharmacy. The collaboration included the exchange of academic information and materials, provision of Clinical Clerkship training at the Clinical Establishment (UHWI in this case), and the provision of academic staff (Clinical instructors, tutors) for support to the programme. The agreement also involved support for integration of education and training in the work environment and cooperation of all members of the Health Care team in the conduct of the programme. The initiative was designed to prepare a cadre of UTech faculty for leadership roles in the planning, implementation and delivery of future offerings of the programme (UTech–UOD Agreement, 2004). (Appendix 11 (a–b) – a) MOU and b) Draft Collaboration Agreement).

Four candidates from the University Hospital of the West Indies enrolled in the Certificate/Diploma/Master of Science in Clinical Pharmacy programme offered at the University of Derby in Academic year 2004/2005.

Arising out of collaborative discussions with The Ohio State University in early 2004, graduates of UTech, Jamaica's pharmacy programme were accepted into the Non-Traditional PharmD programme (NTPD). The programme was designed for licensed practicing pharmacists. At the end of the didactic component of the programme, the candidates were required to engage in clinical rotations in a variety of practice settings. This experience afforded the opportunity for candidates to apply theory, skills and knowledge to pharmacy practice, essential to the formation of quality pharmacists. Faculty of the UTech, Jamaica's School of Pharmacy were contracted to serve as preceptors for the clinical rotations (Memo, January 2004).

In 2013 a Reciprocal Agreement was drafted between the University of Florida, Board of Trustees, Gainesville, Florida, and the University of Technology, Jamaica, to embark on a student exchange programme between the two institutions. The collaborating institutions agreed to make possible the exchange of students between the two universities on a continuing basis (Draft Reciprocal Agreement, 2013). Even though the agreement was not signed officially, in February 2013, a candidate from the first PharmD cohort completed two, 5-week Clinical Rotation Specialties under the University of Florida/Shand's Hospital experiential programme.

University of the West Indies, Mona, Jamaica

Contribution to Course of Study delivery came through the Pharmacology Department, where Mr Paul Singh delivered the contents of the Toxicology module to the Post Diploma students. Mr Singh had a long history of collaborative teaching with CAST, as he was one of the first lecturers to teach Pharmacology in the Diploma curriculum.

University of Houston

In 2004, Dr Sunny Ohia, Dean, College of Pharmacy, University of Houston, held discussions with Mrs Carol White, Dean, Faculty of Health and Applied Science, University of Technology, Jamaica for the drafting of a Memorandum of Understanding (MOU) between the two institutions. The objectives of the MOU which was later prepared included training, education, research and publication activities for the benefit of the respective institutions (Appendix 12 (a-b) – a) MOU between UTech, Jamaica and University of Houston, b) Donation letter and cheque).

PROGRAMME DEVELOPMENT, DELIVERY AND EXPANSION – PHARMACY PROFESSIONALS

During the early years of the transition from Diploma in Pharmacy to the Post Diploma Bachelor of Pharmacy offering, there was the need for additional faculty with specialized training to support several modules which were introduced in the curriculum. The major areas included Pharmaceutical Technology, Clinical Pharmacy & Therapeutics and Toxicology.

Support for the delivery of the Clinical Pharmacy & Therapeutics module came primarily from Doctor of Pharmacy professionals from the United States of America. Most of these individuals were Jamaicans who saw this as an opportunity to give back to their country. One of the patriotic pharmacists is David West, Clinical Pharmacist employed to the CVS Pharmacy chain, who has continued his relationship with the UTech School of Pharmacy for over twenty years. Dr David West visited UTech, Jamaica for four consecutive years (1999–2002) during the summer months. The delivery of the Therapeutics module was conducted over a 10-15-day intensive period.

Dr West also assisted in identifying and recommending other pharmacy colleagues to contribute to the delivery of the Therapeutics module. The quality of the delivery in the Course of Study would have been compromised in those early days had it not been for the contribution of these dedicated pharmacy professionals. Other pharmacists who joined Dr David West to teach the Therapeutics module over the years were Drs Dorothy Brown, Maurice Fuller and Carissa Walker.

Dr David West has continued his relationship with the School of Pharmacy at UTech, Jamaica. In May 2018, he was the Motivational Speaker to the Graduating Pharmacy Class of 2018. His speech was well-received by the students.

The Pharmaceutical Technology module was delivered in a similar intense way by distinguished Professors of Pharmaceutics from Colleges of Pharmacy in the United States or practitioners from the Pharmaceutical Industry. Among the contributors to the Pharmaceutical Technology module were: Loyd V. Allen, Jr., PhD, Professor and Chair, Department of Medicinal Chemistry and Pharmaceutics, College of Pharmacy, The University of Oklahoma. It is worthy of note that Professor Allen is one of the authors for the book, *Pharmaceutical Dosage Forms and Drug Delivery Systems*, published by Lippincott Williams and Wilkins and which has gone through several revisions. The latest edition was published in 2013.

COLLABORATION FOR PROGRAMME QUALITY ASSURANCE

Quality Assurance is all of those attitudes, actions, systems, procedures and objects, which, through their existence and use ensure that appropriate academic standards are attained, maintained and enhanced, in and by the programme, institution or system. The academic standards are made known to the educational community and the public at large. It is a continuous process of evaluating the quality of a higher education system, institutions and programme (UCJ, October 2017).

External Examiners

Since the inception of the Bachelor of Pharmacy degree, the University of Technology, Jamaica has utilized a system of External Examination to assure the relevant standards are maintained for programme delivery and assessment.

The involvement of External Examiners ensures that the institution's awards are comparable in standards to awards granted and conferred by other institutions of higher education. Their comments on assessment procedures, the standard, content and development of the course form a vital part of the processes within the University for the evaluation and monitoring of its courses. The External Examiners also fulfill an essential role in ensuring that all assessments are in accordance with the approved assessment regulations, justice is done to the individual student, and appropriate consideration is given to individual students' extenuating circumstances (UTech, Jamaica Policy on External Examiners for Taught Programmes, Regulations 4, 2017/2018).

Since 2003, the Bachelor of Pharmacy has been externally examined by distinguished Professors of Pharmacy Schools and Colleges in North America and the United Kingdom. Some professors who have served in this capacity have been Professor Peter Redfern (2003–2007), Department of Pharmacology, Bath University, Professor Peter York (2010–2012), Professor of Physical Pharmaceutics, Institute of Pharmaceutical

Innovation, University of Bradford, United Kingdom. Commencing in 2009, the College invited External Examiners with Clinical Pharmacy and Pharmaceutical Sciences specialization to broaden the scope of the review. Since that time, External Examiners with the specific specializations have visited or conducted the review in alternate years. Associate Professor Stephen Pass, Clinical Associate Professor, Texas Tech University Health Sciences Center and School of Pharmacy, Dallas/Fort Wort Campus, USA, served between 2009–2011, a period which overlapped the term with Professor Peter York.

Professor Christianah Adeyeye, (2013–present), Professor of Pharmaceutics and Drug Product Evaluation, Roosevelt University College of Pharmacy, USA, and Professor Rebecca Sleeper (2014–present), Clinical Associate Professor, Texas Tech University Health Sciences Center, College of Pharmacy, Lubbock, Texas, USA have conducted the reviews serving as External Examiners in alternate years (COHS External Examiners' Reports, 2006/7; 2007/8).

Pharmacy Course Advisory Committee

Course Advisory Committees play an important role in the educational process. They are designed to ensure that courses and instructional methods are of high quality and remain relevant. The committee has the task of reviewing an existing course or planning a new course designed to meet identified training needs. Members of the Course Advisory Committee who are representatives of the employers and industry/professional sectors are appointed by the Academic Board. The life of the Committee is three (3) years and this three-year term is renewable (Policy on Course Advisory Committees, 2008/A/11/58A).

The Pharmacy Advisory Committee is comprised of ten to fifteen members appointed by the Academic Board through the Dean. The members are drawn from the Ministry of Health, Pharmaceutical Services Division, Educators, the Pharmaceutical Society of Jamaica, the Pharmacy Council of Jamaica, Pharmaceutical Industry and Employers. Membership shall also include international representatives, who provide comments on specific issues, as well as on broad policy matters. Additionally, recent graduates and representative of the current course student body make up the complement.

Some specific areas in which the Committee contributes include (Policy 2008/A/11/58A):

1. make recommendations and offer advice regarding learning outcomes, the curriculum and the learning environment, in respect of equipment, facilities, and supplies, co-operative education, work experience and placement opportunities needed to optimize the student's learning process
2. to evaluate courses on a periodic basis at least once per year to recommend improvements and/or revisions, as well as analyze reports concerning students' progress
3. ensure that wider national, societal and professional interests are reflected in the University's training courses.

Scholarships and Grants

Support of Pharmacy education for Jamaican pharmacists has been received from government as well as private pharmaceutical agencies and professional organizations. This support has been in the form of Scholarships and Grants to study locally and internationally. Among the sponsors have been the Ministry of Health, National Health Fund (since 2003) and the Caribbean Association of Pharmacists.

Ministry of Health

From as early as the nineteen sixties, the Ministry of Health has offered scholarships to students in the Pharmacy Course of Study at all levels. In some instances, priority was given to those students in level 3 and 4 (years 3 and 4 of the four-year Course of Study since 1996). Beneficiaries must maintain a B average, be a Jamaican citizen and willing to be bonded for 1–5 years depending on the level of support received.

During the 1960s to 1970s, Mr Lester Woolery, Director of Pharmaceutical Services at the Ministry of Health, was instrumental in the establishment of an academic programme with the United Kingdom which saw several persons benefiting from training to the Bachelor of Pharmacy degree in the United Kingdom (CPN, August/Sept 1999).

National Health Fund

The National Health Fund (NHF) was established in 2003 under the National Health Fund Act. Through the Fund, some pharmacists have been trained both at the undergraduate and graduate levels in Pharmacy.

Caribbean Association of Pharmacists

The Caribbean Association of Pharmacists has provided support for educational activities through the UTech, Jamaica Association of Pharmacy Students (UTAPS) over the years. Support has also been given for Leadership and Professional Development initiatives through the UTech, Jamaica Pharmacy Alumni/CIPPPAR organization.

The Afzal Abdool Student Leadership Scholarship was named in honour of the late Afzal Abdool, an esteemed and committed member of CAP. Recipients of the award receive sponsorship to attend the Conference in the year of the Award and to present a collaborative research. At the CAP Conference of 2016, the recipients were Pharmacy students from the UTech, Jamaica (Appendix 13a-b – Students' Reflections).

For the CAP Conference 2019, sponsorship opportunity for Pharmacy students to attend the 2019 Convention in Orlando, Florida, has been advertised. It is anticipated that several applications will be submitted in anticipation of selection for this offer.

University Hospital of the West Indies

Scholarships to study pharmacy have been granted over the years to staff members and their children for entry qualification as well training up-grades. Bonding for a period of time is usually part of the contract agreement.

Pharmaceutical Society of Jamaica

The need to support the training of pharmacists to alleviate the shortage in the profession in the late 1980s was recognised by outgoing PSJ President, Grace Allen, who proposed that private sector companies be encouraged to sponsor the training of pharmacy students, who would then be bonded to serve for a number of years (Allen, 1990). The Pharmaceutical Society of Jamaica has made its contribution to Pharmacy education over the years by awarding students with Grants and Bursaries towards tuition and books. The Society has also recognized Academic Excellence through the granting of Awards at the Faculty/College's Annual Awards Ceremonies.

Pharmaceutical Industry

Pharmaceutical Industry Partners have played their role in the training of pharmacists through the granting of Scholarships, Bursaries and Grants to persons who qualify under the stated criteria for these awards. Consideration for the Award is usually based on need and/or academic excellence.

CIPPPAR/UTech Pharmacy Alumni (UPA)

CIPPPAR and UPA have contributed through the refurbishing of a classroom and the awarding of Grants. There is an annual event to recognize and present awards.

The Vernon Robinson Sr. Memorial Scholarship Award for Academic Excellence was inaugurated in 2018. The first recipient of the Award was Lori-Ann Webb.

UTech Pharmacy Alumni – Canadian Chapter

The Annual Janadian (Jamaican/Canadian) Pharmacist Book Grant was conceptualized in February, 2016.

Other Contributors

Several Pharmacists and Pharmacy owners have given their support to the training of pharmacists through monetary grants and awards, book donations and mentorship. In October 2000, the Dudley Arlington Memorial Scholarship was introduced. To be eligible for this scholarship, applicants should satisfy the following criteria: be in the third year of pharmacy training at UTech, Jamaica, must have a B average or greater that year. The successful applicant would be required to sign a bond to work with Haughton's Pharmacy for a minimum of one year on completion of study. The scholarship provided financing of 50% tuition fees as well as relevant allowances (Mortar & Pestle, 1999–2000).

9.

Leaders/Trailblazers for Pharmacy Education in Jamaica

"History is for human self-knowledge . . . the only clue to what man can do is what man has done. The value of history then, is that it teaches us what man has done and thus what man is."

—*R.G. Collingwood*

The accomplishments we celebrate in pharmacy education today, are the product of hard work, sacrifice, determination, vision and purpose of so many stalwarts, who over nearly six decades, have generated ideas that influenced change and brought about the developments we are proud beneficiaries of in this generation.

This chapter highlights a selection of pharmacy professionals and academic leaders who have played important roles in lobbying for programme development and advancement, or who served as managers, programme developers, programme directors or academic instructors on the journey from apprenticeship to graduate studies in pharmacy.

PRE-INSTITUTIONALISATION PERIOD

Individuals who mark this significant period are those who lobbied to have the training of Pharmacy move from the hospital environment into an academic institution. Worthy of note are members of the professional association whose advocacy to the Governments and Health Ministers of that period resulted in the advancements during the Pre-institutional era. Among the pioneers were stalwarts such as Lester Woolery, Mallman and Strein, Vin Bennett, Vernon Robinson Snr., Jeff Thompson and George Corrie.

INSTITUTIONAL PERIOD

The training of Pharmacists was transferred to the College of Arts, Science and Technology in 1962 in the Science Department. The first Pharmacy Department Head was Bernard Towlson. Haughton (2018) remembered Mr Towlson as a British National who was hired by CAST from his previous educational posting in Ghana, West Africa. Some lecturers for that first class of students were Hopeton Gordon (Zoology and Pharmacognosy), Mrs M. Bruce, (the Art of Dispensing), Irena Cousins (Physiology), Keith Morrish (Pharmaceutics) and Henry Lowe (Pharmaceutical Chemistry).

Mrs Barbara Trewick, Mr Vaschol Scantlebury, Mrs Carol White, Dr Henry Lowe and Dr Riley-Miller, were educators who provided the framework for a sound academic foundation in institutional training of pharmacists between the 1960s and the 1970s.

During the second decade of pharmacy education at CAST, 1971–1980, the key personnel (primarily educators) were Yvonne Crichton and Hugh Lunan (Programme Coordinators), Henry Lowe and George Roper (Heads of Department) and Valerie Kerr (Programme Coordinator).

The period 1981–1990 had as its most outstanding accomplishment the award of the Kelloggs Project Grant and the introduction of the Multidisciplinary Bachelor of Health Science degree. Individuals who must

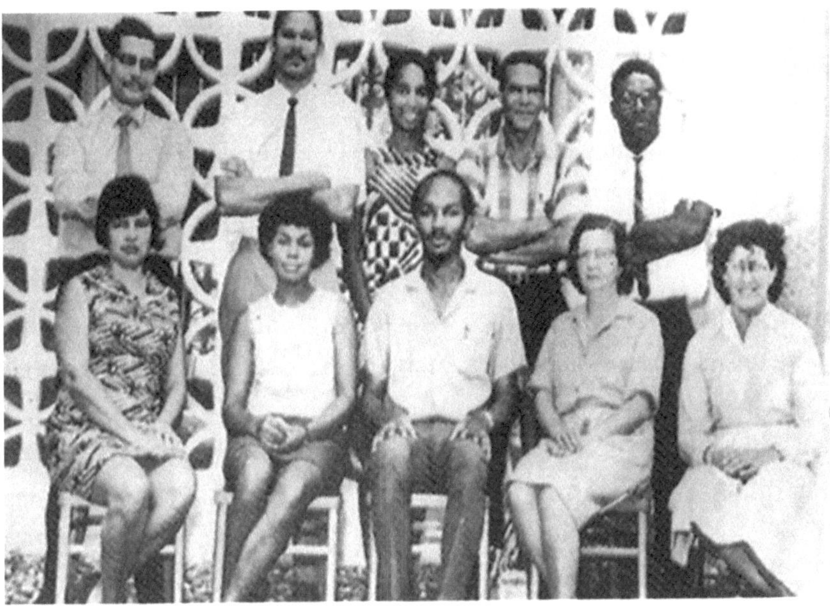

Figure 9a. Early staff of Pharmacy Programme (in the 1960s)

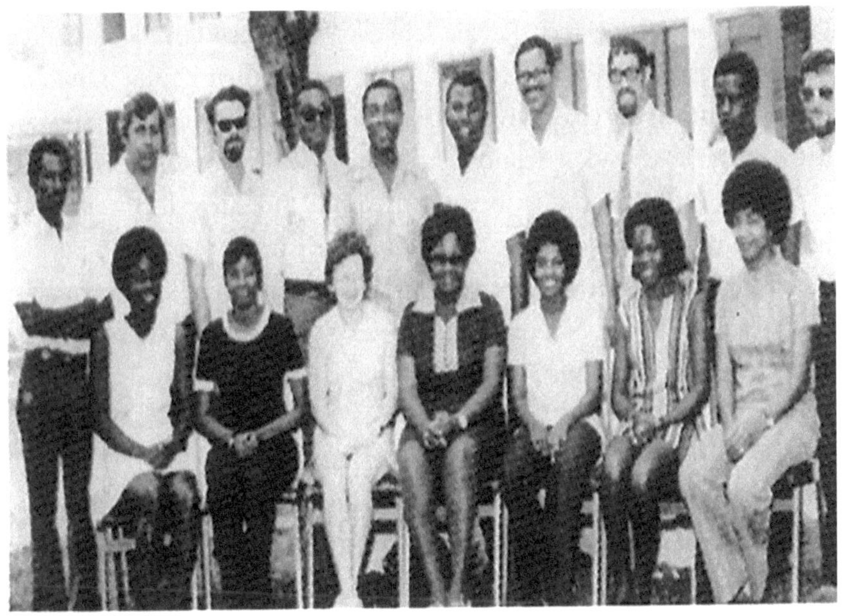

Figure 9b. Early staff of Pharmacy Programme (in the 1970s)

be credited for those significant milestones were: Keith Blayney, Consultant to the Kelloggs Project, Chandra Chennabathni (Pharmacy Programme Coordinator), Harry Drayton (Regional PAHO Project Manager) Eugenie Brown (now Eugenie Brown-Myrie), (Head of Health Sciences Division), Hugh Dixon, and Grace Allen-Young who served in different capacities as Pharmacy educators, while Henry Harris, Keith Golding, Vin Bennett, Lloyd George Logan, Diane Robertson, Donnot James were professional and regulatory leaders who continued to lobby at the Ministerial, Professional Association and Academic Institutional levels for upgrading of the academic qualifications.

The 1991–2000 decade may be considered the most successful years in Pharmacy Education as it was marked by the introduction of the Four-Year Full-Time Bachelor of Pharmacy and Post Diploma Bachelor of Pharmacy degrees. Pharmacists who were instrumental in making the dream of a Bachelor of Pharmacy degree at UTech, Jamaica a reality were leaders from the Professional and Regulatory sectors of Pharmacy at that time. Shown in a 1995 picture from the launch of the Bachelor of Pharmacy degree at UTech, Jamaica are Ellen Campbell-Grizzle (President of PSJ), Thelma Nelson (Chairman, PCJ), Grace Allen-Young (Director, Pharmaceutical Services Div. MOH) and Eugenie Brown now Eugenie Brown-Myrie) (Head of School, Pharmacy) (See Appendix 14).

Other individuals who spearheaded the development and implementation of the degree curriculum were in the 1995–2000 period: Janet Campbell-Shelly, Calvern Bushay, Erin Lun (Canadian Pharmacist /Lecturer), Miriam Naarendorf, Newarklyn Richards as pharmacy educators, and Granville Forbes (PCJ Chairman), C. Aleen Gray, Henry Harris, Grace Muir-Hector and Vivienne Watson (PSJ Presidents), and Yvonne Johnson-Reid (Hospital Pharmacist).

During the 2001–2010 decade the focus was on consolidation and improvement of the programme offerings. Educators and professional leaders who continued the efforts were: Sarafadeen Adebayo, Eugenie Brown-Myrie, Janet Campbell-Shelly, Dawn Lewis, Sean Moncrieffe, Marcia Williams, Juliette Gordon, Andrea Daly, Paul Ellis and Nerissa

Lawrence-Reid. They made contributions to training of the pharmacy students. Lester Woolery and Thelma Nelson (PCJ Chairs), Paul Lindsay, Rosemarie Bailey, Verna Edwards, Vivienne Watson, Norman Dunn served as Presidents of the Pharmaceutical Society of Jamaica during that era. Grace Allen-Young and Hermine Metcalfe served as Pharmacy Advisory Committee Chairs over several terms. Some significant achievements during this decade were the development and introduction of the Master of Philosophy (MPhil) in Pharmaceutics and the Doctor of Pharmacy Curriculae as Graduate Pharmacy Offerings.

Present day contributors (2011–present) who have championed the evolution of academic offerings and the maintenance of the quality in the older programmes include Eugenie Brown-Myrie (who rose to the Office of Faculty Dean), Sean Moncrieffe, Andrea Daly, Marcia Williams serving as Programme Directors and Heads of School, Juliette Gordon, Yvonne Johnson-Reid, Stephanie Mullings, Novlette Mattis-Robinson and Lisa Bromfield served in capacities as Programme Leaders and Programme Directors. Other instructors include Nickania Pryce, Princess Thomas-Osbourne (Part-Time), Janice Bunting-Clarke, Tieca Harris-Kidd, Patricia Robinson, Modupeola Abayomi, Tonoya Toyloy, Michelle Russell and Nerissa Lawrence-Reid. Norman Dunn (PCJ Chair), Ellen Campbell-Grizzle, Valerie Germain, Ainsley Jones, Ernestine Watson, have stood in solidarity as representatives from the Pharmacy Council or the Pharmaceutical Society of Jamaica.

PICTORIAL HIGHLIGHTS

Science Department Heads over five decades

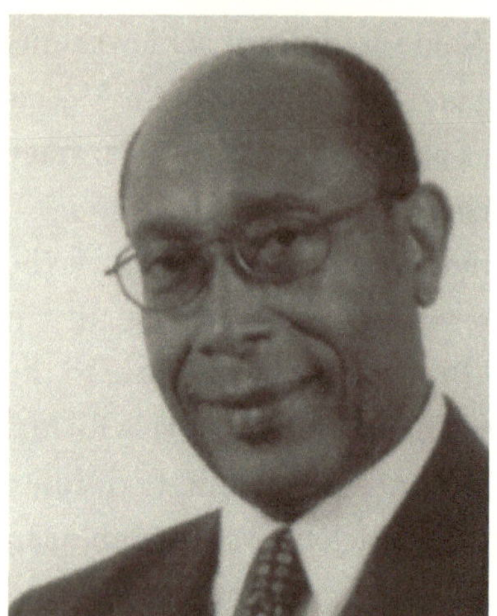

Figure 10. Dr Henry Lowe
(1971–1977)

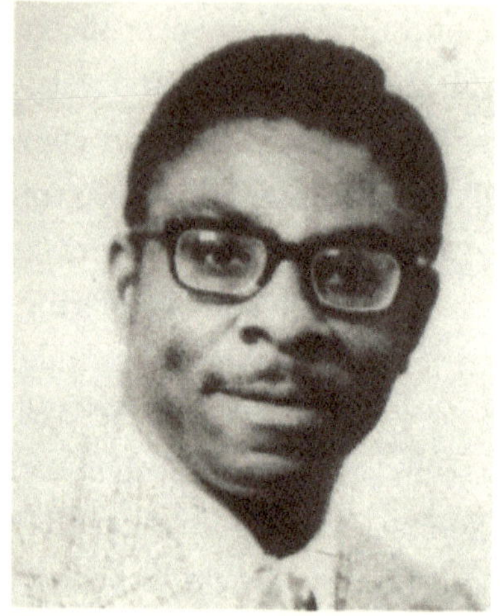

Figure 11. Mr Vascol Scantlebury
(1974–1976)

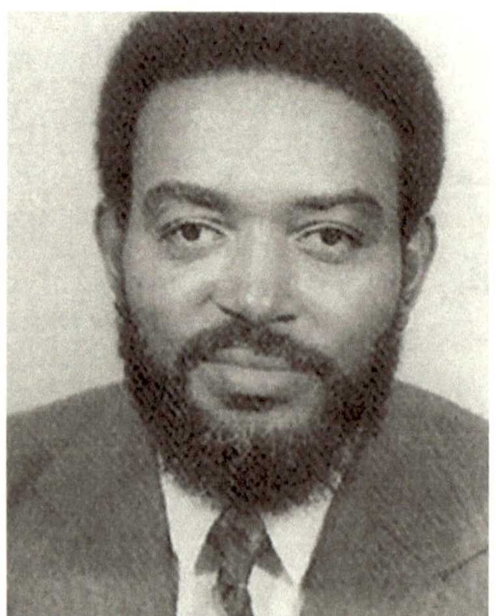

Figure 12. Dr Hugh N. Lunan
(1977–1978)

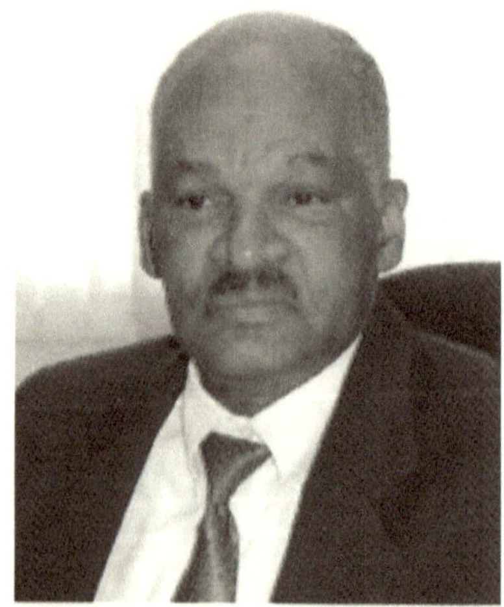

Figure 13. Mr George Roper
(1978–1992)

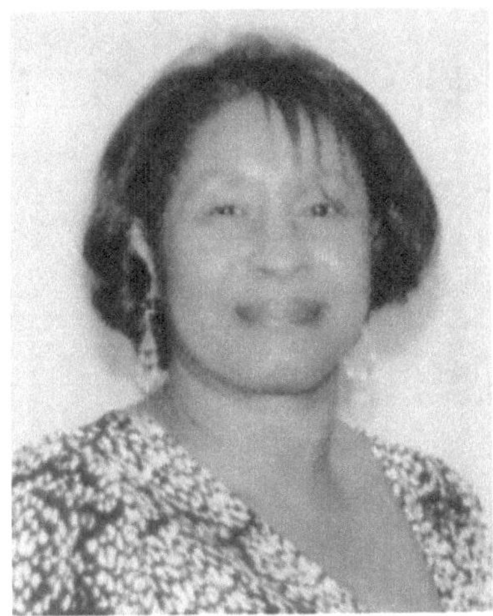

Figure 14. Mrs Carol White
(1992–2007), Dean (1998–2007)

Programme Managers/Directors

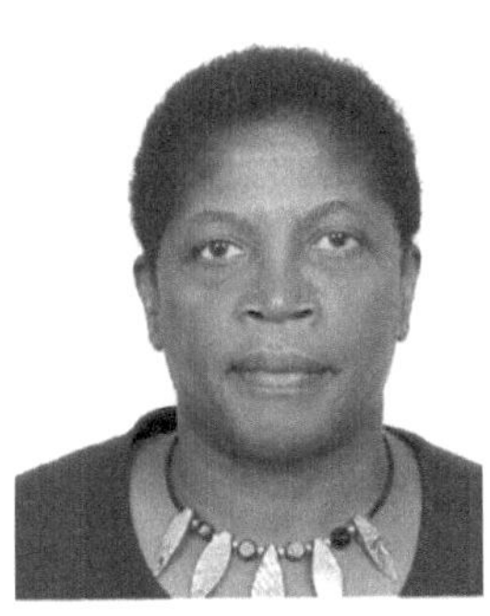

Figure 15: Eugenie
Brown-Myrie, Dean
(2007–2011); Head of
School (2001–2007); Pro-
gramme Director, Doctor
of Pharmacy (2010–2017)

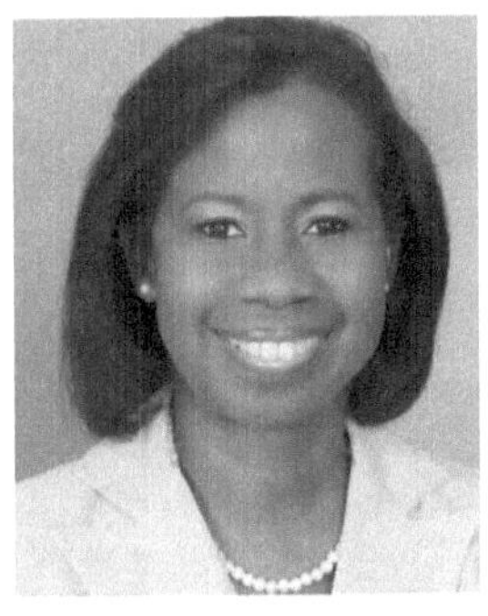

Figure 16. Janet Campbell-Shelly, Dean (2016–
present); Head of School
(2010–2011); Programme
Director (2000–2003;
2007–2009)

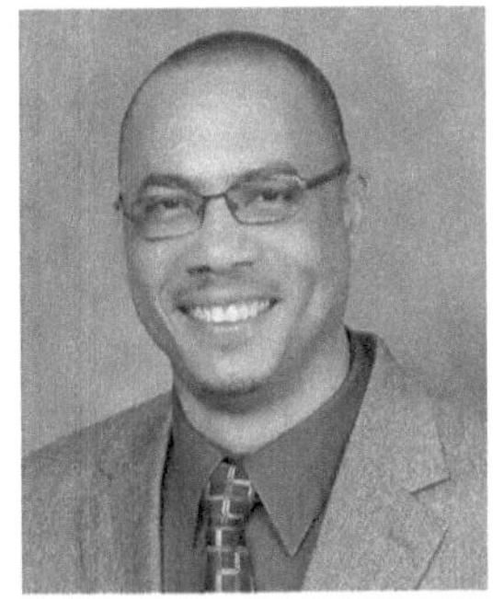

Figure 17. Sean Mon-
crieffe, Head of School
(2011–2016); Programme
Director (2009–2011)

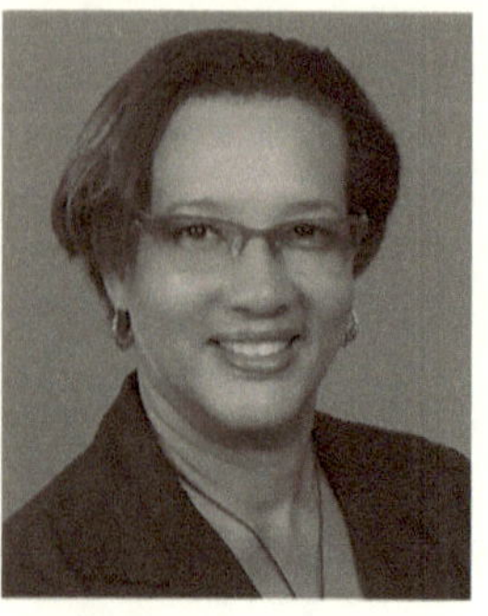

Figure 18. Dr Andrea Daly, Head of School (2016–present); Programme Director (2011–2016)

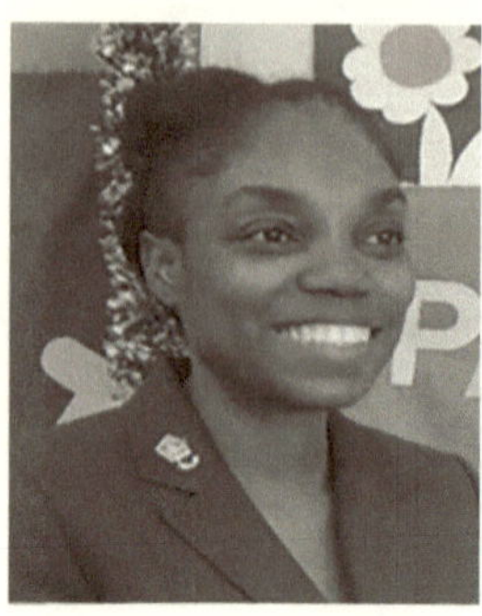

Figure 19. Dr Stephanie Mullings, Programme Director (2016–present)

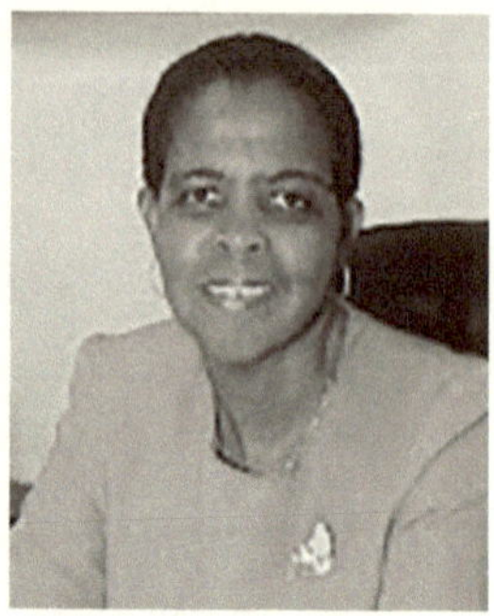

Figure 20. Dr Marcia Williams, BPharm. Programme Director (2004–2008), PD Bachelor of Pharmaceutical Technology (2014–2018), PD MPhil/PhD Pharmaceutics (2018–2020)

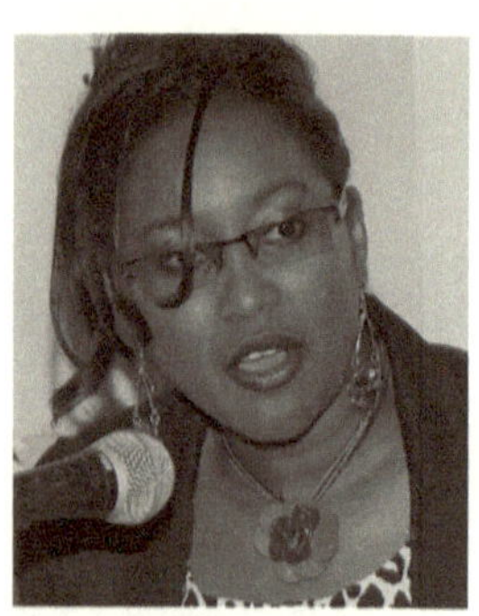

Figure 21. Mrs Tieca Harris-Kidd, Programme Director, Bachelor of Science Pharmaceutical Technology (2018–present)

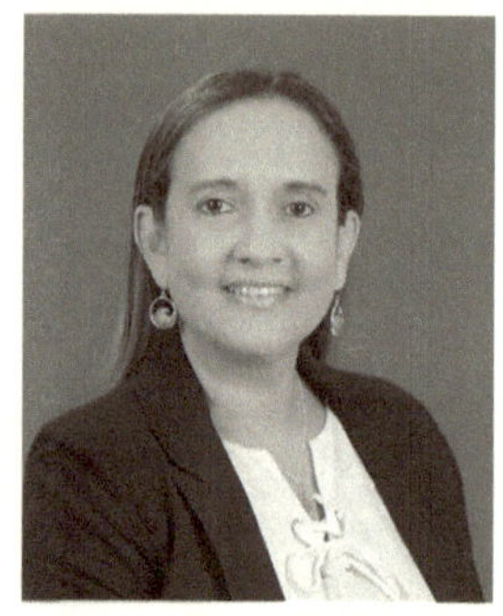

Figure 22. Dr Lisa Bromfield, Programme Director, Doctor of Pharmacy (2017–present)

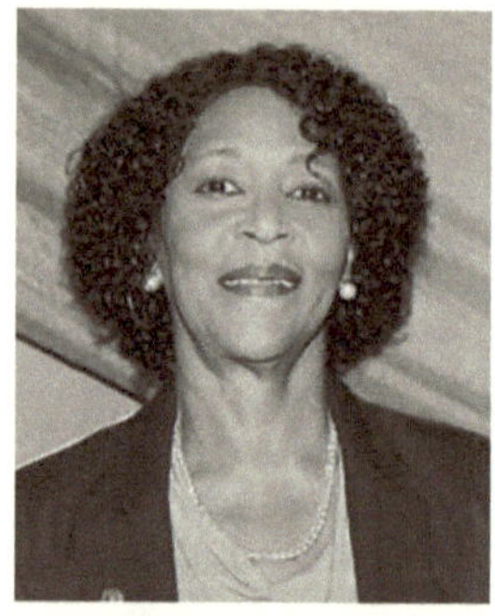

Figure 23. Mrs Yvonne Johnson-Reid, Programme Director, Pharmacy Technician Course of Study (2009–2016)

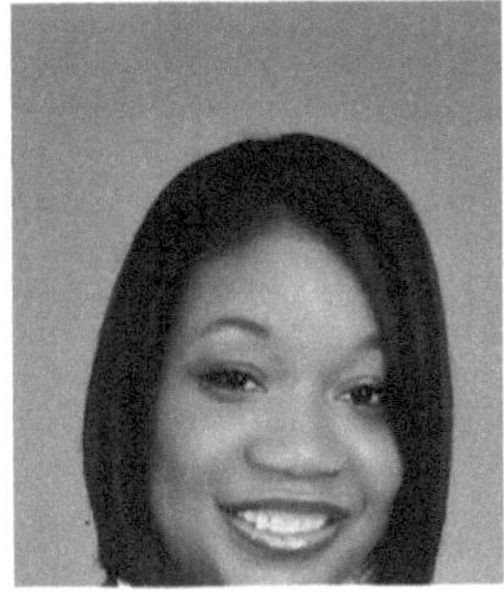

Figure 24. Miss Nickania Pryce, Programme Leader, Pharmacy Technician Course of Study (2018–present)

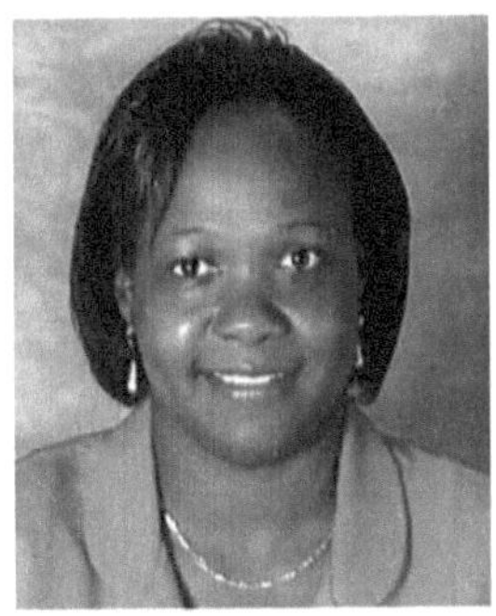

Figure 25. Mrs Novlette Mattis-Robinson, Programme Director, Online Post Diploma Pharmacy (2013–2018)

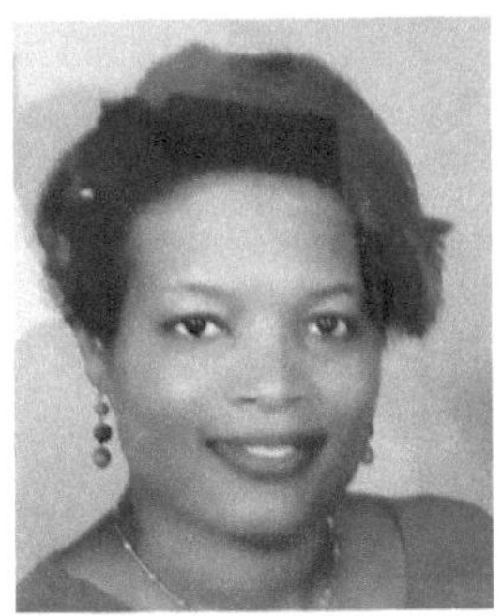

Figure 26. Dr Janice Bunting-Clarke, Programme Director, Online Post Diploma Pharmacy (2018–present)

Programme Highlights

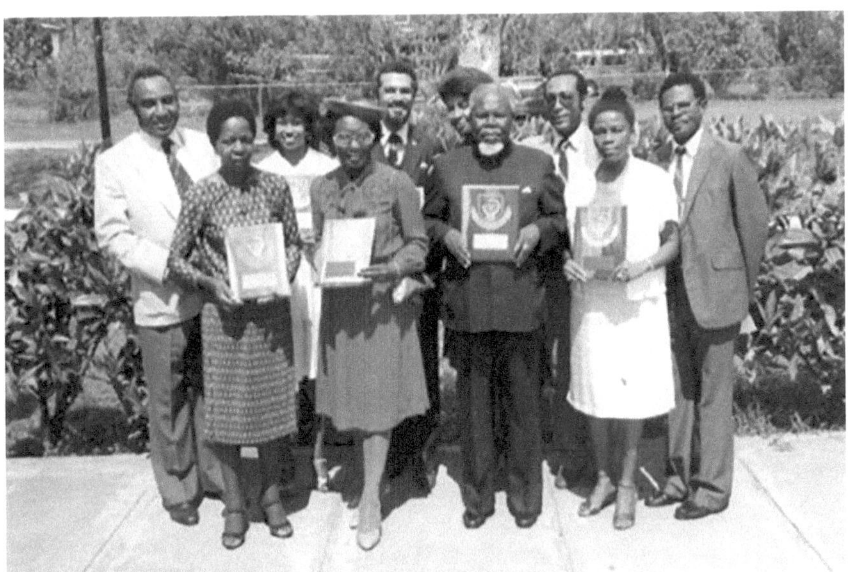

Figure 27. Pharmacy Pioneers at 21st Anniversary Celebration of Pharmacy Programme at CAST (1983)

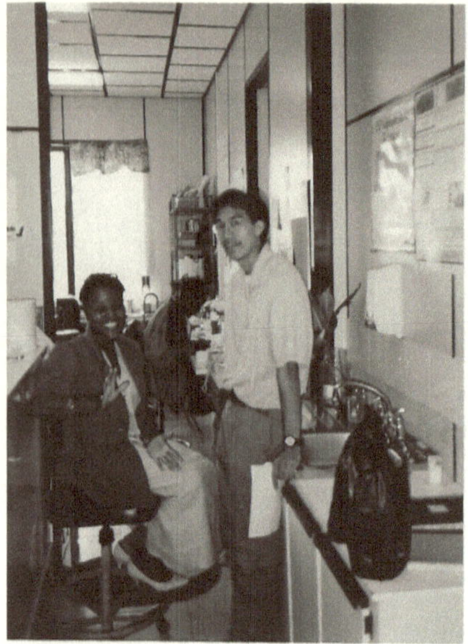

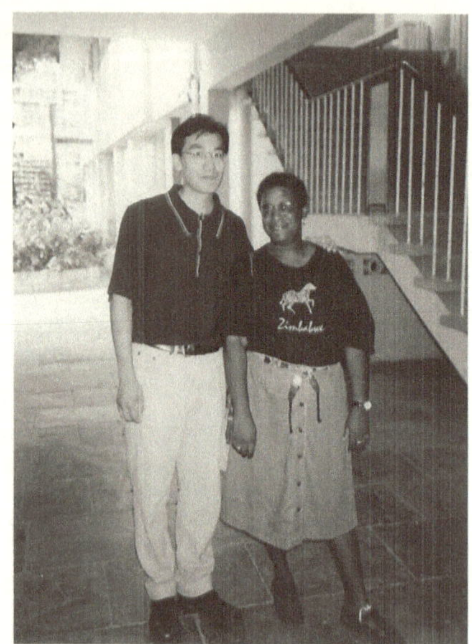

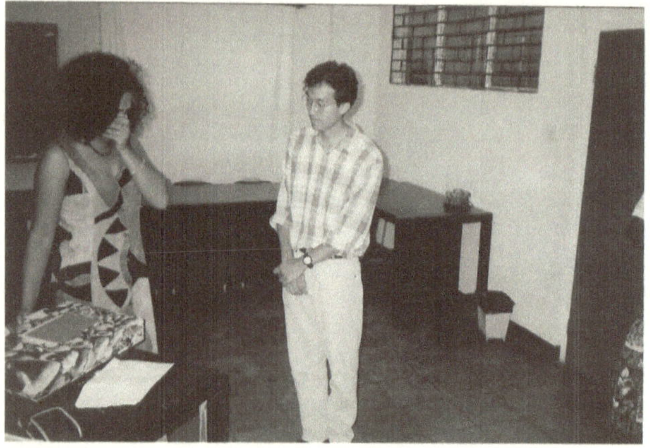

Figure 28. Eric Lun, Canadian Pharmacist and Lecturer, instrumental in the development of B.Pharm. curriculum

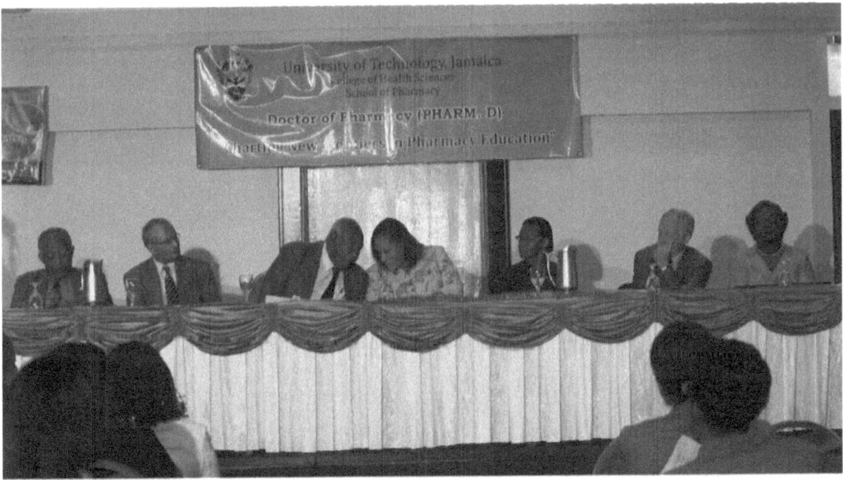

Figure 29a. Head Table at Launch of Post Baccalaureate Doctor of Pharmacy (PharmD) programme (2010)

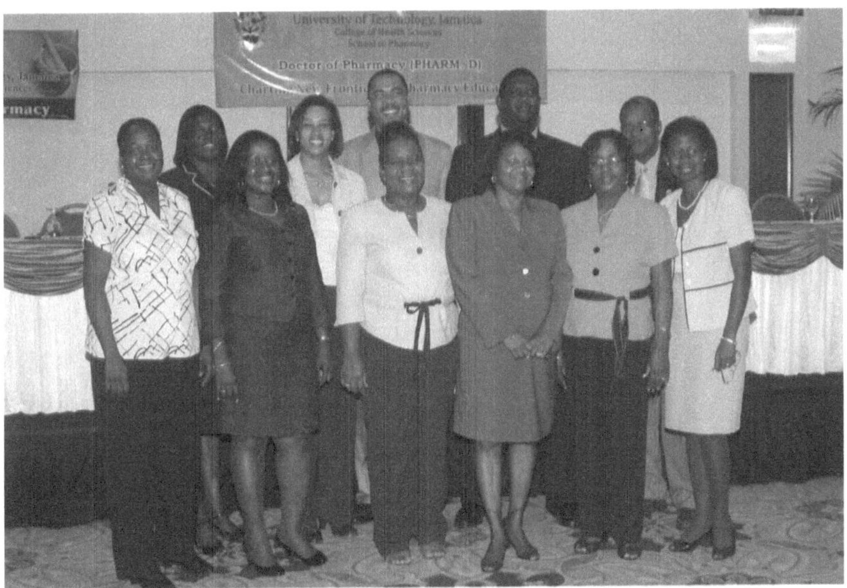

Figure 29b. COHS staff at Launch of Post Baccalaureate Doctor of Pharmacy (PharmD) programme (2010)

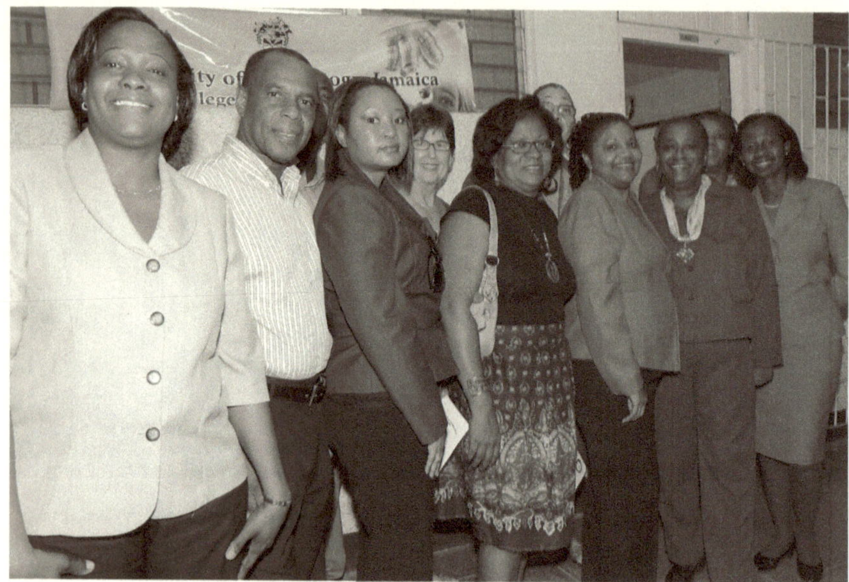

Figure 30. Launch of Online Post Diploma Bachelor of Pharmacy degree programme

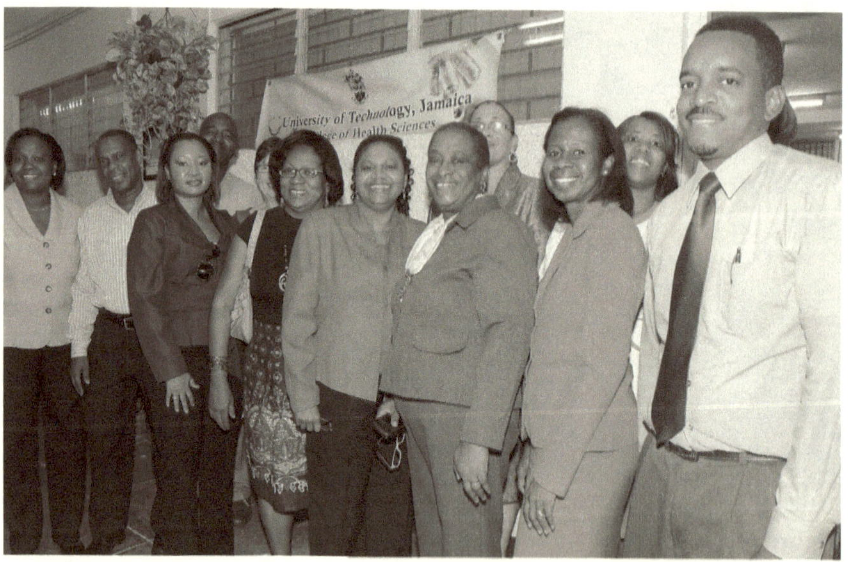

Figure 31. Caribbean Stakeholders at Launch of Online Post Diploma Bachelor of Pharmacy Course of Study (2013)

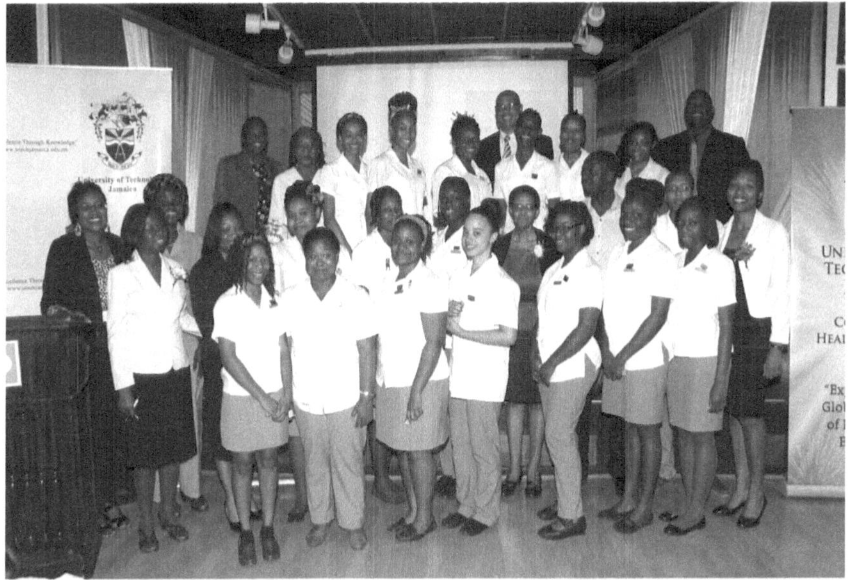

Figure 32. Launch of Bachelor of Pharmaceutical Technology degree programme (2015)

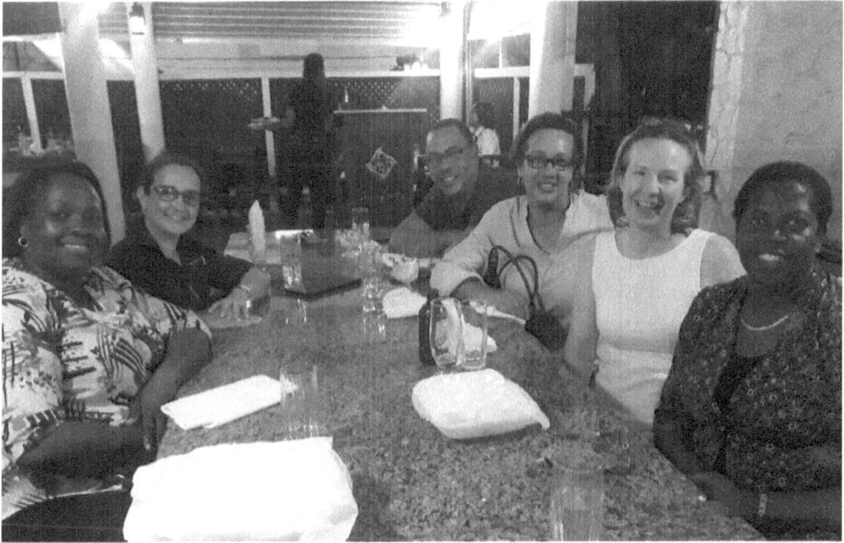

Figure 33. Facilitator and participants for Bedside Training, 2018

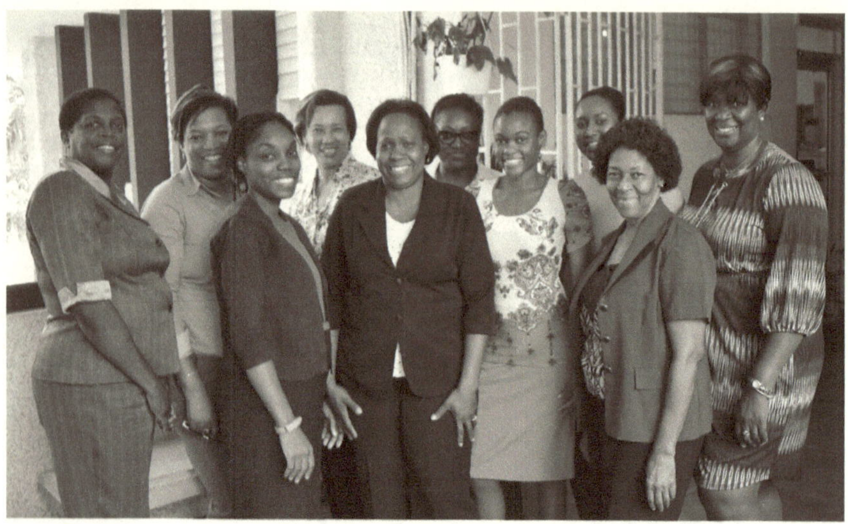

Figure 34. Some UTech Pharmacy Managers and Lecturers in 2019

Student & Graduate Highlights

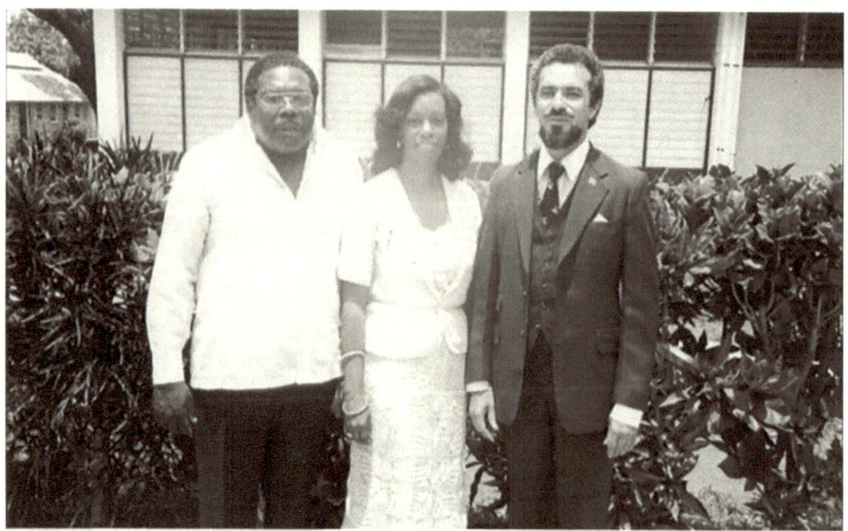

Figure 35. Graduates from 1st batch of CAST Rx Students – Vin Bennett Jr, Stafford Haughton & Joan Melbourne Neill

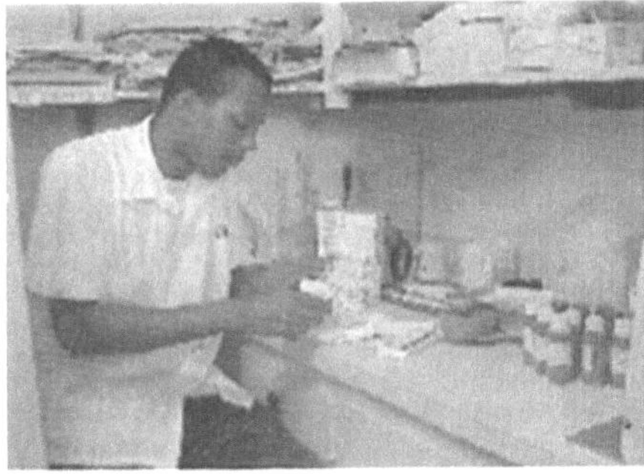
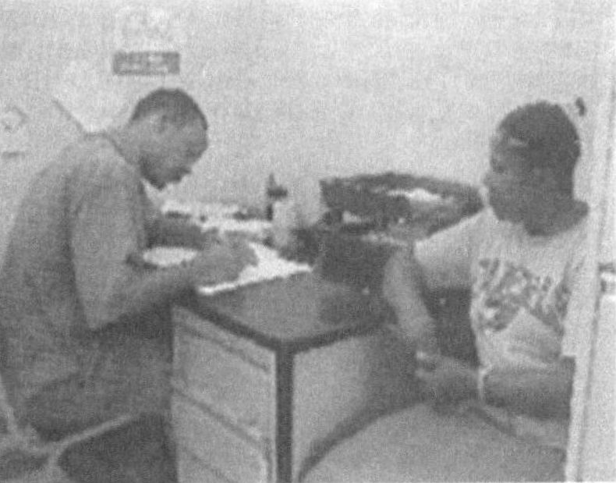

Figure 36. B.Pharm. students showcase their skills at Faculty Open Day, 2002

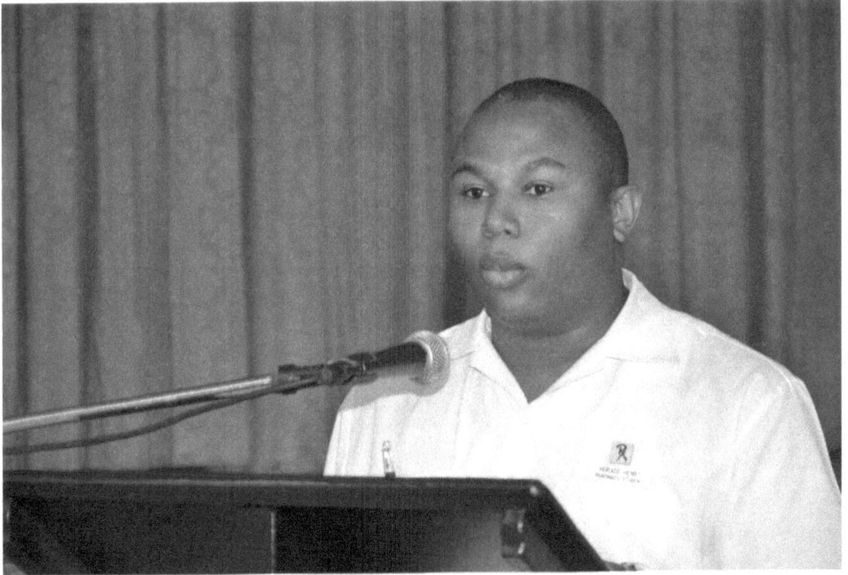

Figure 37. Horace Henry, University of Technology Association of Pharmacy Students (UTAPS) President 2011–2012

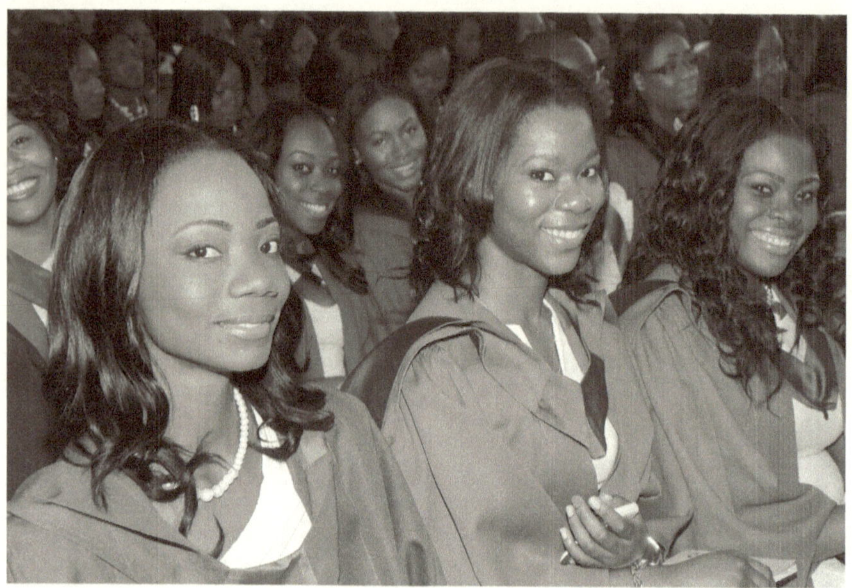

Figure 38. B.Pharm. students at Graduation, 2013

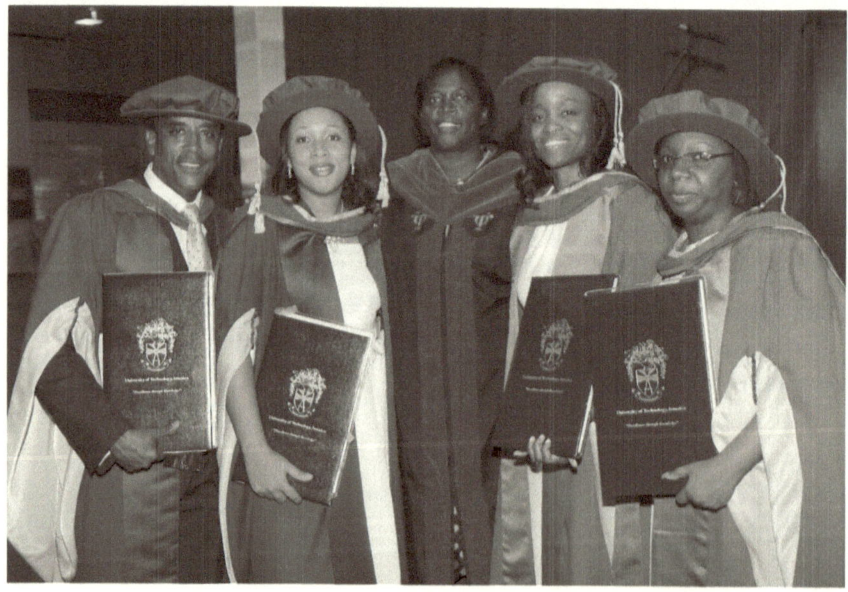

Figure 39a. Graduates of First Cohort of Doctor of Pharmacy candidates, (2013 in Kingston)

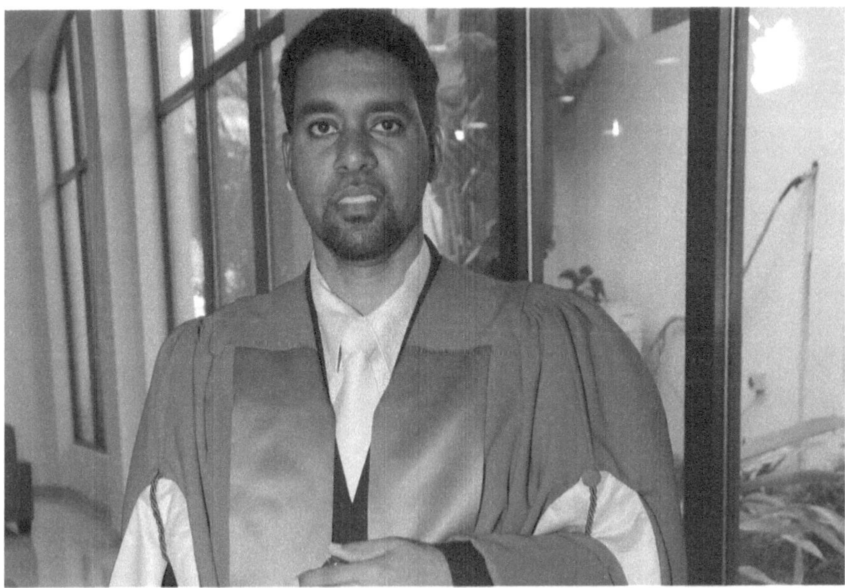

Figure 39b. Cleston Headley, Graduation of First Cohort of Doctor of Pharmacy candidates (2013 in Montego Bay)

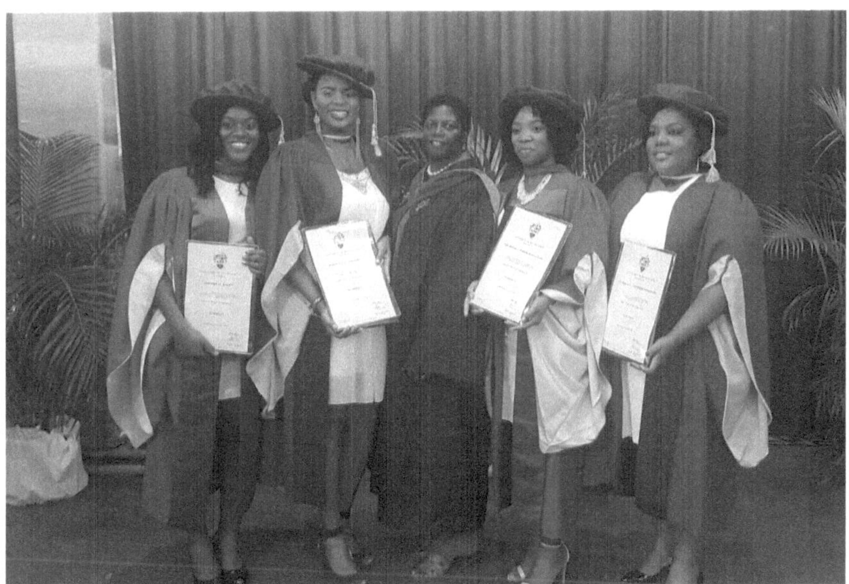

Figure 40. Graduates of Second Cohort of PharmD candidates (2016)

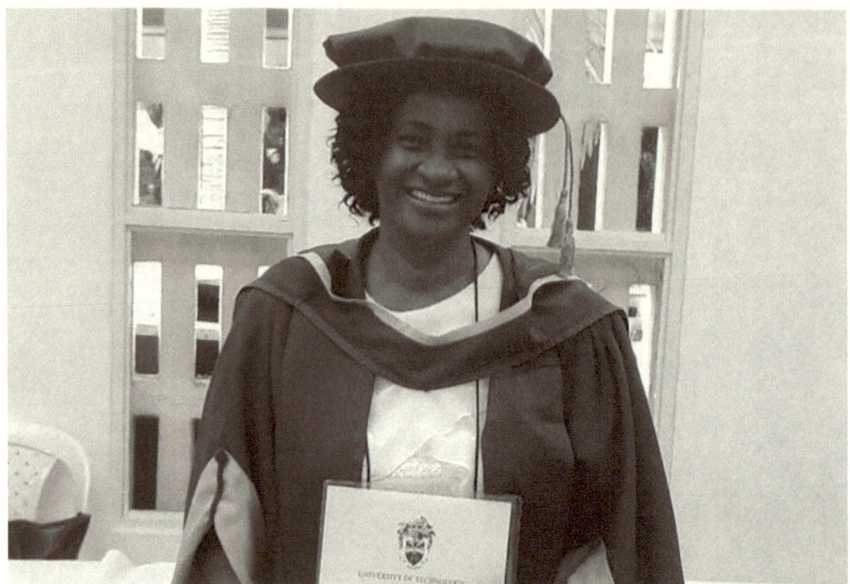

Figure 41. Rose Victory Evans, Graduation of Third Cohort of PharmD candidates, 2018

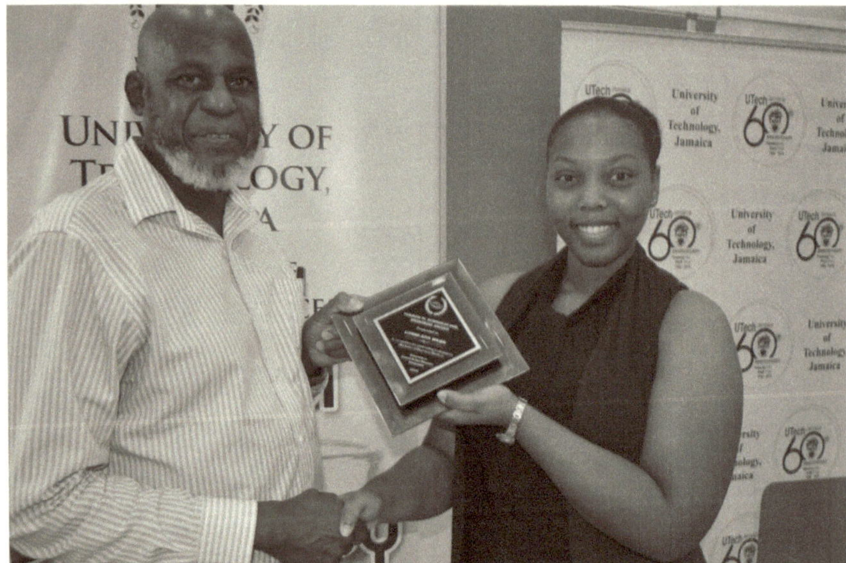

Figure 42. Lori-Ann Webb, Pharmacy Scholarship recipients of the Vernon Robinson Memorial Scholarship, 2018

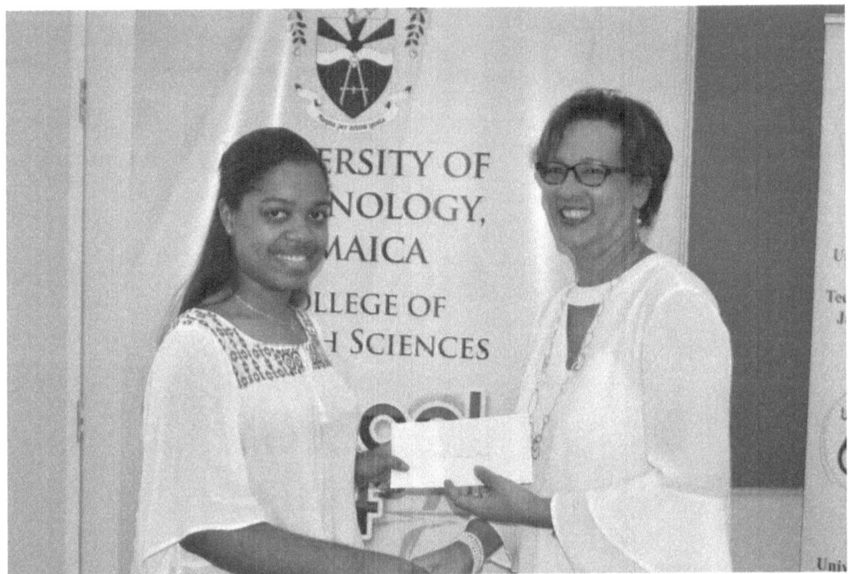

Figure 43. Dr Andrea Daly presents Scholarship cheque to Pharmacy student, 2019

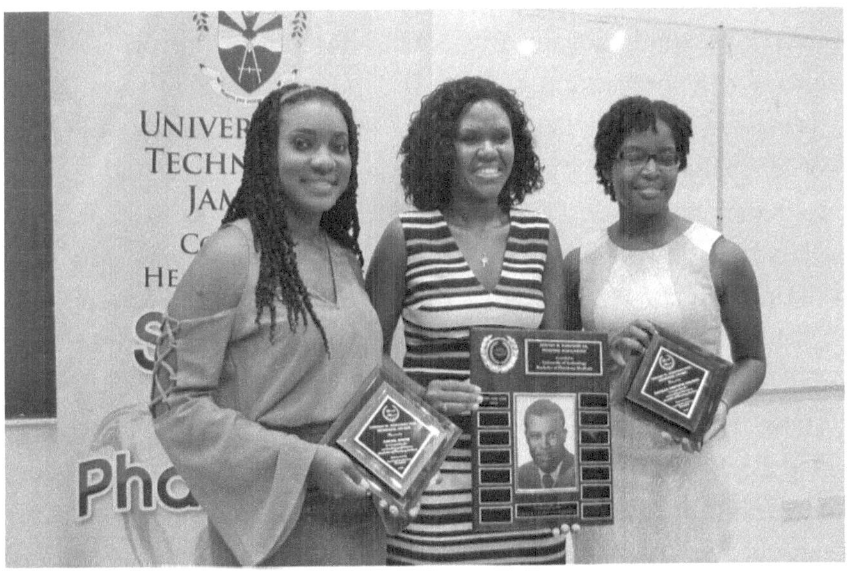

Figure 44. Pharmacy Scholarship recipients of the Vernon Robinson Memorial Scholarship, 2019

10.

Ongoing Advancements in Pharmacy Education
Sharing the Vision

Pharmacy education must remain dynamic, whether at the institutional level or through continuing education/continuing professional development programmes. Over the many decades of the history, Pharmacy Educators, Regulators and Professional Leaders have used various platforms to charge, challenge and motivate pharmacists to engage in academic pursuits that will advance the quality of service to their clients.

Pharmacists were exhorted to redefine their roles and demonstrate the value of their services at a Commonwealth Pharmacy Day Reception as far back as 1999. The then Head of the School of Pharmacy and Health Sciences, Dr Eugenie Brown (now Eugenie Brown-Myrie), in her message as Guest Speaker at the Reception, encouraged pharmacists to operate as integral members of the Health Care Team. She also shared opportunities for Pharmacists in a wide range of practice areas, namely, Self Care Consultants, Drug Information Specialists, Health Educators, Specialist Practitioners, Geriatric Pharmacotherapists, Prescribers and Managers of Chronic Diseases (Common Waves, 1999).

In 2000, Mr Lester Woolery, Managing Director, LASCO Pharmaceuticals Division, writing in *Caribbean Pharmacy News,* appealed to Pharmacists to adopt robust policies to enable the profession to play its rightful role in the changing pharmacy environment. He posited that pharmacists must continually update professional knowledge, embrace and manage change, while lobbying for relevance in training programmes. As members of the health care team, pharmacists need to increase involvement in health promotion and preventative medicines and market themselves as a profession that spans the boundaries between health and social care. He ended his appeal by stating that, "each of us has the opportunity to be an architect of Pharmacy's future. I put it to you that the future of Pharmacy is in your hands" (*CPN* vol. 2# 4 July/Aug 2000).

New Business Opportunities – Sports Medicine was a feature article that appeared in *Caribbean Pharmacy News* in 2003, suggesting that pharmacists should develop the requisite expertise and offer valuable services to athletes. The Editor intimated that the pharmacist can become a very important resource person for addressing doping in sports, assisting athletes and coaches to make the right decisions in the selection and use of medications and nutritional supplements. She emphasized that pharmacists have unique knowledge of pharmacology and therapeutics, making them ideally placed to advise on permitted substances and permitted routes of administration (CPN, March/April 2003). Pharmacists may therefore carve out their own niche in another practical area through specialized training in the area of Sports Medicine. The opportunities for pharmacy are endless.

Many voices have echoed their support, not only for the pharmacist in educational achievements and service provision, but also in recognition of the pharmacy technicians whose roles and responsibilities have resulted in the removal of some routine functions from pharmacists so that they can be available to deliver more advanced patient care services.

President of the Pharmaceutical Society of Jamaica, Mr Henry Harris, in a 2004 article in the *Society's Retreat Magazine* shared his vision for the role of the Pharmacy Technicians. He expressed the view that the Pharmacy

Technician group should be included in the Pharmacy Regulations. This move would give recognition to this important group of professionals for education, certification and monitoring of the practice. He advocated that Pharmacists and Pharmacy organisations should collaborate with Regulatory authorities to ensure that regulations governing the certification and utilization of Pharmacy Technicians are compatible with the support of the pharmacist in the provision of direct patient care. He opined that Pharmacy Technicians should be innovatively used as a means of achieving the goal of increased pharmacist involvement in direct patient care activities (*Harris PSJ Retreat Magazine*, 2004).

In 2008, Mr Lester Woolery as Chairman of the Pharmacy Council of Jamaica (PCJ) made reference to the enlarged professional responsibilities which opened new professional opportunities. He outlined job opportunities in the UK to emphasize his stance on the matter (Woolery, 2008). UTech, Jamaica graduates were challenged to seek broader horizons in becoming specialists in new areas of pharmaceutical practices. Mr Woolery's advocacy continued into 2009. In his article entitled "Career Paths in Pharmacy" Mr Woolery outlined "Paths to the future".

PATHS TO THE FUTURE

In his discourse, Mr Woolery, articulated that the future of Pharmacy does not lie behind a dispensing counter. Many pharmacists have gone into Management, Business Administration and Marketing, while making ample use of their pharmaceutical experience. There are areas of specialization, which have attracted interest and have seen pharmacists completing postgraduate courses in: Oncology (Cancer) Management, Cardiology Management, HIV/AIDS Management, Diabetes Management, Public Health, Regulatory Pharmacy, Infection Control, and Paediatric Pharmacy. These varied areas of practice will see the long-awaited change in the face of pharmacy coming to fruition (Woolery 2009).

The Pharmaceutical Society of Jamaica (PSJ) must be commended for the expanded portfolio of the Continuing Education Committee in 2009-10. The new committee, called the Continuing Education and Training Committee (CET) was established to a) provide educational activities to enable members to keep apace of advancements in science and modern concepts of pharmacy and b) to facilitate the training of pharmacists in an effort to broaden the scope of pharmacy and to contribute more holistic care to patients. The CET Chair reported that training focus would include Outreach, Therapeutics and Professional/Personal Development. Other suggested areas were: Basic cardiac life support, Diabetes Education, Public Speaking, HIV/AIDS Counseling and Testing, Asthma Educators, Immunization and Tobacco Cessation (Reid, 2017). The future of pharmacy will be determined by the pharmacy professionals' motivation and ongoing desire to improve the health services to persons who need to access the care. Improvement in health care is best achieved through collaborative practice paradigm; members of the health care team using a multidisciplinary approach to provide the care. At the International Pharmaceutical Federation (FIP) Centennial Conference in 2012, conference speakers shared important approaches to achieving improvement in Health through responsible medicines use. Some ideas included creating multidisciplinary teams of physicians and pharmacists for improving quality and safety in medication use, incorporating interdisciplinary education in the health professions and establishment of regulatory framework for collaborative practice in the context of scope of practice and accountable care. Other areas that were discussed at the Conference were better drug therapy management, improved patient care outcomes, impact of technology in pharmacy practice and pharmacy practice research (FIP Centennial Preliminary Programme, 2012)

Another visionary gave his challenge in 2016. "What we in Jamaica and the Caribbean see as future trends in pharmacy practice is already a reality in more developed countries. Worldwide, pharmacists have evolved, diversified, specialized and upgraded to remain an important and integral part of the healthcare team (Dunn 2016). Dr Dunn expressed the view that with regional universities having expanded their training to the professional doctoral level, the foundation is laid for Caribbean pharmacists to position themselves for the global shift. (*PSJ/CAP Conference Magazine*, July 2016).

The authors are heartened by the fact that Dr Dunn, Chairman of the PCJ has taken on the challenge to convince Regulators and Health Professionals to accept the new roles. This process would begin with lobbying for the amendment of the Pharmacy Act and Regulations as well as the Public Health Act (*PSJ/CAP Magazine* July 2016). We wish him and the rest of the new PCJ team, which has the vision of taking the practice of pharmacy in Jamaica into the 21st Century every success.

PSJ President Ainsley Jones shared in 2017 that the PSJ would be placing focus on Geriatric Pharmacy in order to enable seniors to maintain the best possible health (Jones, 2017) PSJ Conference Magazine June 2017).

THE VISION REALISED

A robust Continuing Education Programme accredited by the Pharmacy Council of Jamaica is one of the achievements of the Pharmaceutical Society of Jamaica and other providers delivering cutting edge information relevant to the pharmaceutical industry. Continuing Education linked to Annual Re-registration of Pharmacists was enacted in 2003 and is now embraced by all pharmacists.

Amendments to The Pharmacy Act, 1975 to include Pharmacy Technicians are currently under consideration for enactment. This will see the Pharmacy Council having responsibility for regulating the training, Registration and monitoring of the practice of this group of Pharmacy Support personnel.

Currently, training for several practice specializations has been initiated in UTech programmes as well as through short Certification courses or Continuing Education Credits provided by the Pharmaceutical Society of Jamaica, Ministry of Health and other providers of Continuing Education. For example, training in Diabetes Education and Management, Contraceptive Technology, Asthma Management, Tobacco Cessation, Pharmacy Immunization, Basic Life Support, HIV/AIDS Counselling and Testing, and Guidelines for the Care and Treatment of Persons with HIV Infection, are some specialization areas where pharmacists have identified practice niches.

The academic programmes in pharmacy in Jamaica have incorporated formal experiential training, which presents the opportunity for learning and practice in a multidisciplinary health care environment, both at undergraduate and graduate levels. These programmes include the full-time Bachelor of Pharmacy and the Post-Diploma Bachelor of Pharmacy at the undergraduate level and the Post Baccalaureate Doctor of Pharmacy (UTech PharmD Curriculum, 2009) and Entry Level PharmD at the University of the West Indies, Mona (UWI PharmD Curriculum, 2016).

New on the horizon is the Ministry of Health's recognition of Clinical Pharmacists, with the establishment of Clinical Pharmacists' posts in hospitals. Currently four Clinical Pharmacists are employed and assigned to Type A, B or Specialist Hospitals in Kingston and St Andrew, Mandeville and Montego Bay.

In tandem with the mushrooming of Pharmacy Specializations is the impending review and amendments to Acts and Regulations to impact the provision off expanded pharmacy services.

VISIONS NOT YET REALISED

Pharmacists are yet to embrace in a significant way, the business opportunities that may flow from Sports Medicine and Geriatric Management.

BARRIERS TO IMPLEMENTATION OF VISION AND POSSIBLE SOLUTIONS

The provision of pharmaceutical care and its associated pharmacy services requires requisite training, competence and motivation, all of which involve a heavy investment of time and resources. Many professionals are frustrated in their efforts to provide a greater level of pharmacy services to clients. An important way of addressing this challenge would be to use Pharmacy Technicians to complement the role of the pharmacist and optimize patient outcomes. This was a recommendation made by a former PSJ President, Henry Harris in 2004.

Coupled with the time limitations, the availability of flexible and accessible training courses and financial affordability are other obvious barriers to the realization of some vision ideas.

SUGGESTIONS FOR THE FUTURE

Pharmacy and healthcare education must continuously strive to stay ahead of the changes occurring in relation to healthcare delivery and management. Therefore, as we prepare students for their future roles and assist practicing professionals in their development, the pharmacy curriculum as well as CE and CPD programmes must seek to address the current and future healthcare needs of the patients and the wider society. Following up from the list of unrealized visions as well as keeping abreast of changes and trends, some areas which must be considered to improve pharmacy education and practice are: Financial support for education and training, patient safety, geriatric care, impact of technology on practice, herbal and alternative medicines, medicinal marijuana and regulatory changes necessary to ensure high standards of practice. Additionally, considerations should be given to emerging diseases based on the impact of environmental pollution and climate change.

Many students who obtain places to study pharmacy are unable to support their education and training because of lack of financial support. Pharmacy industry partners, Pharmacy alumni associations, financial aid programmes at the universities, government agencies and non-governmental organisations must begin or continue to establish Scholarships and Grants that can provide the needed assistance to many of these bright minds who can become assets to the profession and nation. Bonding agreements may be considered in some of these arrangements.

The ultimate goal in the provision of pharmacy services is to achieve optimum outcomes in patient health and wellbeing. To achieve these goals, pharmacy education and practice should include a focus on patient safety issues with an emphasis on reducing medication errors, adopting pharmacovigilance measures and eliminating counterfeit medicines from the market.

The demographics for the present day patient population are showing an increasing shift towards the elderly. The geriatric patient experiences pharmacodynamic and pharmacokinetics changes which influence their response to use of drugs. As such, academic institutions and providers of pharmacy education and continuing education must continue to revise curricula and CE offerings. This should include the introduction of specialized training that will keep pharmacy students and pharmacists on the cutting edge of medication management in the geriatric patients.

Technology has brought so many changes to the way we provide services and how we communicate with our stakeholders. It is of utmost importance that pharmacy practitioners obtain the requisite basic and ongoing technology training in order to keep abreast of computer programmes and other technological devices that can be used to enhance the practice of pharmacy. On a regular basis, practice guidelines and policies, clinical research findings and new product information are introduced via scientific databases. The practitioners need to become aware and knowledgeable about how to access and use the information appropriately. The advent of social media provides an enhanced avenue to communicate with patients about pharmacy services and medicines management.

Electronic prescribing is becoming a reality in Jamaica. It is the secure electronic generation, authorization, and transmission of a prescription between an authorized registered practitioner and a registered pharmacy of choice (Cox, 2016). The system of transfer introduced should be authentic, and ensure integrity, security, and confidentiality of the transaction. In order to ensure these processes are maintained, the necessary legal and regulatory framework must be in place. This requires the collaboration of several stakeholders, primarily, medical and pharmaceutical professions and relevant Government agencies. At the centre of this service is the patient, whose rights to privacy, confidentiality, access to information and freedom of choice should not be violated.

The Amendment to the Dangerous Drugs Act in 2015 decriminalized marijuana and legalized the use of medicinal marijuana. This has resulted in the establishment of new agencies/authorities with regulatory responsibilities for cultivation, manufacturing, distribution and dispensing of medicinal marijuana. These developments have created the need for training of pharmacists to ensure compliance with the Pharmacy Act & Regulations, Food and Drugs Act and Regulations and other legal instruments which guide the proper dispensing, sale and use of marijuana products. Additionally, the developments have also provided opportunities for policies, guidelines and other such publications to be generated for dissemination in a Public Education Campaign.

11.

Considerations for Future Academic Directions

PHARMACY RESIDENCIES AND FELLOWSHIPS

Pharmacy Education offerings in Jamaica have expanded to include the Bachelor of Pharmacy, Post Baccalaureate Doctor of Pharmacy (UTech, Jamaica) and Entry Level Doctor of Pharmacy degrees (UWI). The authors believe the time has come for the institutions offering pharmacy studies to develop and deliver post graduate courses with either a clinical or research focus. Residency programmes are post graduate training with a clinical focus, while a research focus training is referred to as fellowship programmes. In keeping with the identified opportunities for pharmacy practice, UTech, Jamaica and UWI should consider developing Residency and/or Fellowship programmes in areas such as: Geriatric Pharmacotherapy, Oncology, Cardiology, HIV/AIDS, Endocrinology, Infectious Diseases, and Paediatric Pharmacotherapy.

PHARMACY SPECIALIZATION COURSES

Some pharmacists may not be desirous of pursuing programmes for an extended period of time after their undergraduate studies. They may be given the opportunity to enroll in short courses in specialisation areas of their choice. These courses would be delivered over several weeks or months and would serve to enhance their practice. Shorter courses may be offered in any of the areas listed in the previous section as well as areas such as Regulatory Pharmacy, Sterile Technology, Herbal and Complimentary Medicines, Pharmacy Specialization for Sports Injuries and Treatments, or any other identified area of practice. In June 2018, Pharmacists holding Masters and Doctoral degrees in Clinical Pharmacy enrolled in a one-week intense Bedside Training Course delivered by an oversees Clinician and Consultant Pharmacy Practitioner. The training was a combination of classroom and clinical sessions conducted at the University Hospital of the West Indies. Participants were presented with a Certificate of Participation.

PHARMACIST RESEARCHERS

According to Koshmann and Blais (2011), research may be defined as studious inquiry or examination, especially, investigation or experimentation aimed at the discovery and interpretation of facts, revision of accepted theories or laws in the light of new facts, or practical application of such new or revised theories or laws. Pharmacists are competently trained to carry out investigations that will produce findings that add to the existing body of knowledge.

Pharmacists should be involved in all aspects of health research, from basic laboratory investigations to population-based studies.

The Canadian Society of Hospital Pharmacists in a 1995 statement posited that, "any unknown in the practice field is a potential research idea". The Society included the following as research topics for institutional pharmacists:

- basic pharmaceutical sciences, including the development and testing of new dosage forms or medication-administration modalities

- clinical research concerning the efficacy, safety, and pharmacokinetics of drugs
- pharmacy practice research addressing various issues such as the evaluation of new and existing services, workload measurement, pharmaco-economics, and quality management (CSHP, 1995)

These are all appropriate areas that Jamaican pharmacists may consider doing as they establish themselves as pharmacist researchers.

CONTINUING PROFESSIONAL DEVELOPMENT

Continuing Education is defined by the Accreditation Council for Pharmacy Education as a "structured educational activity designed or intended to support the continuing professional development of pharmacists and/or pharmacy technicians to maintain and enhance their competence (ACPE, 2007)". Continuing education in pharmacy is typically delivered in the form of lectures, workshops, or written home study materials. It is required by many countries around the world for the renewal and maintenance of pharmacist licensure (Vlasses, 2006). Continuing Professional Development has been defined as "the responsibility of individual pharmacists for systematic maintenance, development, and broadening of knowledge, skills and attitudes to ensure continuing competence as a professional throughout their careers." (FIP, 2002). Contrary to traditional approaches to CE, the most pervasive model utilizes a cycle that encompasses reflection, planning, acting (learning), evaluating and recordings as the key elements of the learning process. Ultimately, it is considered to be a self-directed outcomes-focused approach to lifelong learning (FIP, 2002; ACPE 2014).

It has been widely accepted that CE alone is insufficient for successfully meeting lifelong learning needs of health professionals (Driesen, Verbeke, Simoens and Laekeman, 2011). In the Jamaican setting, CE has become mandatory for annual re-registration of pharmacists. Although pharmacists satisfy this requirement, many seem to lack the interest and motivation and only do enough to satisfy the minimum requirement of 12 CE credits annually (Driesen, et al, (2005).

In addition to using CE as a requirement for professional licensure, Hanson et al, (2007) suggested that other top enablers of CE are personal desire to learn and enjoyment provided by learning as a change for routine barriers to participation. Another study identified most common motivating factors to participating in CE activities as gathering practical knowledge, and keeping scientific knowledge up to standards (Driesen, et al, (2005).

BARRIERS TO CONTINUING EDUCATION (CE AND CPD)

Surveys of Flemish, Quatar and Egyptian pharmacists concluded that the most commonly cited barriers to CE were time, excessive workload, job constraints, cost, lack of programme accreditation and un-interesting subjects (Driesen et al, 2005; Wilbur, 2010; Ibrahim, 2012). Other documented barriers to CPD are time constraints, lack of resources, lack of motivation and interest, system and technical problems, facilitation and support issues and poor understanding of the CPD process (Donyai et al, 2011).

Reid (2017) reviewed the sensitization efforts towards CPD in the Jamaican setting over the past four decades. From the review she reports the following:

Continuing Professional Development (CPD) has been on the mind and lips of some of our colleagues since the 1970s. Hugh Lunan (1976) referred to it as Continuing Competence of Pharmacy Practice in his article of the same name. To be competent he explained was to possess sufficient knowledge, and ability to meet specified requirements in the sense of being able, adequate, suitable and capable.

Dr Grace Allen-Young in 1999 remarked that she would like to see change from product-focused practice to patient-centered service. She held the vision of the establishment of a Caribbean College of Pharmacy Practice. This, she felt was one way of advancing change through CPD

(Allen-Young, 1999).

CPD was one of the "key planks" articulated by CAP during the deliberations for harmonization of pharmacy legislation in 2005. The crucial role of organized continuing professional development was highlighted. There was lobbying for increased availability of distance education options to support CPD by delegates who attended the 2006 CAP Convention held in St Kitts & Nevis.

Mr John Bell, CPA President, in his message to the CAP/CPA Conference August 2001 stated that, "Education was the key to the profession's future success – education of pharmacists and education of the community by pharmacists". He ended by highlighting the fact that it was essential for pharmacists to maintain the public's trust by continued involvement in Professional Development Programmes (Bell, 1999).

During the period 2010–2014 the Association's Quality and Ethics Committee introduced the CPD concept to the CAP membership. Unfortunately, it only received luke-warm interest. It is good to note that some of our Caribbean Pharmacists see CPD as very important. Margaret Wilson-Blake, a pharmacist at the University Hospital of the West Indies, Mona, Jamaica circulated templates to her colleagues more than a decade ago to promote the concept. Reid (2017) commented on the efforts of the professional colleagues, "I am happy that some of our colleagues have caught the vision and are not only taking personal responsibility for their professional development, but are documenting their advancement".

Mandatory Continuing Education has been a requirement for annual re-registration of pharmacists in Jamaica since 2003. As a result of that regulation, Jamaican pharmacists must complete 12 hours of CE each year to remain on the Register of Pharmacists. With the increasing move towards pharmacists engaging in Continuing Professional Development, it is incumbent on the professional organisations in Jamaica to organize training programmes that will guide pharmacists through the CPD process and enable them to develop the requisite skills and attitudes to participate in the CPD activities. Cross and Tofade (2014) posited that "pharmacists who underwent training in CPD and those using tools to facilitate the process were more likely to use it successfully, thus making the availability of these resources imperative to the expanded implementation of CPD". The authors believe that as a future move to increase participation in CPD, Pharmacy Schools must consider the inclusion of CPD principles in the curriculum so that pharmacy students will be exposed to the concept during their formal pharmacy education year. This early exposure should increase the knowledge of and appreciation for CPD and ultimately expand their involvement in the process.

HARMONIZATION OF PHARMACY EDUCATION AND LEGISLATION

Discussions about harmonization have been ongoing for over three decades. Since 1989, CARICOM has promoted the free movement of personnel throughout the region. Under the Grace Allen-Young Administration (CAP President 1992–94) the Canadian Pharmaceutical Association accessed funding and worked with CAP to complete a preliminary document on Harmonization. This achievement made pharmacy the pioneers of the concept of Harmonization in the region (Reid, 2017). This harmonization aimed to establish a Caribbean Examining Board (CARIPEB).

The proposal for the establishment of a Caribbean Pharmacy Examining Board (CARIPEB) was endorsed unanimously at the Council Meeting of the Caribbean Association of Pharmacists, Hamilton, Ontario on August 27, 1991 (Council Minutes). The Council members then proposed that the countries to constitute CARIPEB were Jamaica, Barbados, Trinidad and Tobago, Guyana and the Organization of Eastern Caribbean States (Brown, unpublished work).

The expected actions for the implementation of CARIPEB were formal endorsement of the concept, resolution to establish CARIPEB, lobbying activities with governments, the public-consumer groups, other health professions and fellow pharmacists (Council Minutes, 1991).

The concept of a Caribbean Pharmacy Examining Board (CARIPEB) received broader endorsement by delegates at the CAP Convention held in Montego Bay, Jamaica in 1992. Later, in 1994 at the CARICOM Health

Ministers Conference the document on Harmonization was accepted. Recommended Guidelines for the establishment of CARIPEB were also approved by the Health Ministers. Despite the early enthusiasm and wide regional support in the initial stages, the establishment of the Board being a next logical step did not materialize. The support from the licensing bodies and CAP which was necessary to get additional Canadian funding was also not forthcoming (Reid, 2017).

The proposed benefits of CARIPEB were considered to be: harmonization of pharmacy qualifications through a single examining body, acceptance by all licensing bodies of the CARIPEB qualification, no reviews or further examinations, portability, no impact on pharmacists already licensed, no "grandfather" clause required, no requirements for changes in existing legislation, no financial impact on governments, and pharmacists who have passed the CARIPEB examination can add the letters "CARIPEB" to their list of qualifications (CAP Council Minutes, 1991).

Although the concept was initially well received among Caribbean pharmacists, its full implementation was never realized. Since Harmonization of pharmacy is still a goal for the region, the concept of a CARIPEB may still be a future initiative. CARICOM agreed to free movement of CARICOM nationals with university degrees in 1995. That decision started the debate regarding the level of pharmacy qualification which should be accepted in the region. Since only persons with degrees could move and work in August 1999 CARICOM Health Ministers emphasized the need for the pharmacy profession to move towards Harmonization in order that professionals could move freely. That recommendation was closely aligned with the CAP agenda: to promote a higher standard of Pharmacy Practice, and hence the need for higher qualification (Reid 2017).

The CAP Convention, Curaçao in 2001 is associated with an important historical milestone for the profession of pharmacy and pharmacy education. At that Convention, the delegates ratified the decision to establish the Bachelor of Pharmacy as the minimum requirement for practice in the region [The "Curaçao Accord 2001"] (Reid, 2017). Pharmacy education in Jamaica and Trinidad had already upgraded to the Bachelor's degree level, both institutions having introduced the four year degree qualification in 1996. Now, in 2018, the University of Guyana and Belize have implemented Bachelor's degree programmes and the University of the Bahamas has trained pharmacists to the degree level through a Franchise Agreement with the University of Technology, Jamaica.

In 2013, UTech, Jamaica introduced a fully on-line Bachelor of Pharmacy degree programme for registered pharmacists in Jamaica and the Caribbean to upgrade their certification from diploma to Bachelor's degree. This on-line offering has attracted applicants from several Caribbean countries, including Belize, St Lucia, Grenada, Barbados and Jamaica. This programme offering has facilitated the upgrading of pharmacists from countries where the development and implementation of the Bachelor of Pharmacy degree may prove challenging for various reasons.

The Pan American Health Organization (PAHO) has supported the efforts of harmonization and has introduced several initiatives to advance the realization of this vision. The PAHO organized a Workshop on Pharmacy Education in the Caribbean in Barbados, May 20 and 21, 2009. The first term of reference (TOR) for that meeting was: **Harmonization on Pharmacy Education.** The stated objective was to develop a proposal for harmonization of pharmacy education, including the profile of a pharmacist in the Caribbean, basic pharmacy curriculum and entry requirements. The activities that would enable the group to achieve the objective were outlined. They included:

a. identification of schools' focal points
b. survey of current programmes (to examine core competencies, core components/courses, entry level requirements, staff and resources)
c. review of proposals from Pan-American Conference on Pharmacy Education (core curricula), PAHO/WHO and other international recommendations and experiences from health professions in the Caribbean

d. liaison with CARICOM for official recognition of model curriculum

e. development of a draft proposal for circulation

f. discussion on possible adaptation and adoption by programmes.

At a PAHO meeting in 2013, the following statement was communicated in relation to harmonization:

> In the Caribbean, pharmacy education programmes have different durations, orientations and lead to different certifications, namely diploma, associate degree, Bachelor's Degree and Pharm D. Except the last one, all professionals are named and registered to practice as pharmacists. In most of the cases, there are no differences in terms of attribution of this professional. Considering both the CSME and the health sector context, adjustments in the pharmacy programmes are necessary (PAHO Meeting 2013).

The Pan American Conference on Pharmaceutical Education for approximately two decades discussed the subject of Harmonization of Pharmacy Education in the Americas. A proposal was drafted in the 1998 conference in Lima, Peru and has undergone revisions in subsequent conferences. Although progress has been made on the curriculum for the **BASIC PHARMACEUTICAL EDUCATION PLAN FOR THE 21ST CENTURY,** the final decision is yet to be made. And so the arguments continue and efforts for harmonization of pharmacy education in the region continue to evade us.

Challenges & Barriers

While we continue to embrace the concept of Harmonization in Pharmacy Education for the Caribbean region, we must keep in clear focus the barriers and impediments that have delayed the progress in the academic sphere. Some challenges or barriers that continue to make harmonization of practice and legislation elude the pharmacy profession in the Caribbean are as follows (Reid, 2017):

• the different levels of education accepted for practice. The Bachelor of Pharmacy is compulsory for practice in some jurisdictions such as Jamaica. Associate degree, Diploma, and Certificates are applicable in some;

- without harmonization, each individual jurisdiction will determine its educational requirement and competency to practice;
- only some pharmacy schools in the Caribbean offer training to the Bachelor of Pharmacy level. Students would therefore have to meet the cost of travel and related costs to access education;
- the reluctance of policy makers and pharmacy leaders to make these big decisions might be due to the fact that practicing professionals as well as training institutions which deliver the courses below the Bachelor of Pharmacy level would be adversely affected.
- finally, higher levels of training and free movement could have an impact on wage relations and availability of human resources.

Regional and International Collaboration

A long list of collaborating organizations exists that have contributed to the development and advancement of Pharmacy Education in Jamaica over the last six decades. The opportunities for ongoing partnerships are endless as we incorporate technology in the educational offerings. Not only can the collaborators assist in education at the undergraduate and graduate level but they can play significant roles in the provision of specialized education and training areas which will facilitate lifelong learning opportunities for pharmacists. Collaborating institutions and consultants accessible globally include International Pharmaceutical Federation (FIP), Pan American Health Organization (PAHO), Accreditation Council for Pharmacy Education (ACPE), universities and individual pharmacy consultant practitioners.

The Memorandum of Agreement between the College of Arts, Science and Technology (CAST), Jamaica and the School of Community and Allied Health, University of Alabama at Birmingham, (SCAH/UAB) was conceptualized in 1983. At the meeting held at the Ministry of Health,

Jamaica on July 5, 1983, Project Hope's Consultant in Allied Health, Dr Keith Blayney, contracted under the Technical Assistance component of the World Bank – Government of Jamaica Loan Agreement, proposed recommendations for linkages with CAST. The recommendations addressed CAST's position with respect to present and future health manpower training needs in Jamaica. Recommendations proposed the establishment of a Department of Health-related Sciences which would incorporate existing Allied Health training programmes within the Science Department of CAST and other non-CAST National Allied Health training programmes. There was also a suggestion to establish inter-institutional linkages between the proposed Department of Health Related Sciences, CAST, and other local and overseas institutions, in order to provide assistance in four key areas: programme development, faculty development, student assistance and administrative/organizational assistance. The linkage agreements should include, among other things, elements of student academic credit transfers to overseas institutions, faculty exchange, faculty training, teaching assistance and funding support (MOA SCAH/UAB and CAST, 1984).

The recommendations were implemented with the development of the Multi-disciplinary Bachelor of Health Science degree, supporting disciplines such as Medical Technology, Pharmacy, and Public Health Inspectors. Other areas of the collaboration that brought benefits to CAST were funding support, faculty training and teaching assistance.

In 1992, Mr George Roper, Head of the Science Department, CAST, and Dr Eugenie Brown (now Eugenie Brown-Myrie), Programme Director, Pharmacy were invited to the Southeastern University of the Health Sciences, Florida, to discuss linkages between the two institutions. From that visit, the discussions included the possibility of having CAST graduates continue their studies at the Southeastern College of Pharmacy (SECOP) to obtain either their Bachelor of Science in Pharmacy (BS) or Doctor of Pharmacy (PharmD) degree. Arising out of the discussions, several CAST graduates received acceptance to Nova Southeastern University Programme of Pharmacy at an advanced level. The primary objective of the collaboration was to have graduates return to the educational institution or country to enhance the clinical and didactic programmes or pharmacy practice, respectively. However, very few pharmacists who continued pharmacy studies at SECOP, did not return to Jamaica; they have been incorporated into the United States Pharmacy practice.

PROFESSIONAL ACTIVISM

Pharmacists are uniquely positioned within health care. They are trained in a wide range of areas: business, management, human behaviour and pharmacology and pharmaceutical science. As such, they can be a source of support for patients at all levels of health care (Marotta, 2017). The time is ripe for pharmacists to operate as social activists, building coalitions, working to promote policies and influence actions that will create awareness and influence social change. Some areas in which pharmacists can engage include advocacy, public education and campaign programmes surrounding counterfeit medicines, accidental poisoning, environment pollution and waste management, domestic violence, drug abuse, among the long list of social factors that impact on one's health and wellbeing. Activities that pharmacists can get involved with as part of their activist role, may be through the following areas: https://www.acs.org/content/acs/en/careers/college-to-career/chemistry-careers/social-impact.html

- communication with policy makers, business leaders and community organizations through publications, speeches, public events or media
- research the effects and implications of factors that negatively impact health and wellbeing.
- organize responses to disaster and environmental degradation
- formulate position statements, goals and priorities for campaigns
- track environmental changes, environmental pollution in Jamaica
- work towards improving standard of living among marginalized communities through financing health programmes, education and technology from developed nations.

CONCLUSION

Pharmacy Education in Jamaica has evolved from a simple apprenticeship programme to a sophisticated highly structured and formalized academic system over more than a century. Current practitioners have benefited from the work of visionaries and educators who have contributed to the advancement of Pharmacy Education in Jamaica. The authors now challenge the current practitioners to be a part of the change process, to continue the advancement, maintain professional practice standards in keeping with international trends and realize future goals conceptualized by the Visionaries and Pharmacy Leaders.

Appendices

Appendix 1: Certification Letter for a graduate of the 3-year course of Study at the end of the KPH era

DRUGS AND POISONS CONTROL BOARD,

MINISTRY OF HEALTH ANNEXE,

35 NORTH STREET,

KINGSTON,

IN CASE OF REPLY PLEASE QUOTE THE
DATE OF THIS LETTER AND THE FOLLOWING

No. DB/76

29th April, 19 62.

TO WHOM IT MAY CONCERN

THIS IS TO CERTIFY THAT ＿＿＿＿＿ ＿＿＿＿＿ ＿＿＿＿＿ pursued a course of study in Pharmacy for a period of three years and satisfied the Board of Examiners at the Qualifying Examinations held on the 26th, 27th & 28th October, 1962, in the following subjects, the pass mark being 60% :-

SUBJECTS		MARKS
Pharmaceutical Chemistry	-	71%
Orals	-	75%
Pharmaceutics & Materia Medica	-	78%
Forensic Pharmacy	-	82%
Practical Dispensing & Idents	-	65%

She was granted a Druggist's Licence on the 24th. April, 1962.

CHAIRMAN

DRUGS & POISONS CONTROL BOARD.

I, the undersigned, hereby certify that the foregoing document is a true copy of the original thereof.

Signed at Montreal, Quebec, October 19, 1970.

PIERRE L. CARON, NOTARY.

Appendix 2: Accreditation of Bachelor of Pharmacy Degree

Accreditation of Bachelor of Pharmacy degree

The highpoint in pharmacy in Jamaica in the past six months was the accreditation of the Bachelor of Pharmacy degree by the University Council of Jamaica. The degree programme is offered by the University of Technology has three entry options:

1. A four year programme open to persons who have two 'A' levels in addition to five 'O' Levels or CXC Caribbean Examination Certificate that include English, Mathematics, Chemistry, Biology and another science subject preferably Physics;
2. a three summer modular Post-Diploma programme open to Diploma who have at least two years working experience as a pharmacist;
3. a one-year full-time programme open to persons satisfying the same conditions named in #2 above.

The interest of practicing pharmacists to upgrade their education is phenomenal with current applications being approximately four times the number of available spaces!

The University is now challenged to offer the Masters degrees in pharmacy. It however is in need of clinical pharmacists and would welcome interested persons to contact:

Dr Eugenie Brown, Head of School of Pharmacy & Health Science, 237 Old Hope Road, Kingston 6, Jamaica [Tel: (876) 917-1699].

Submitted by - Mrs E. Grace Allen Young
CPA Vice-President

Source: CPA Newsletter May 2001- Number 63

Appendix 3: Letter to Mr Lester Woolery – Re Contract for Clinical Training

```
26 November, 1990


Mr Lester Woolery,
Director of Pharmaceutical Services,
Ministry of Health,
10 Caledonia Avenue,
Kingston 5.

Dear Mr Woolery,

The contract for delivery of the Clinical Pharmacy Orientation
Programme is now subject for renewal for the 1990 - 91 year.
However, there is need for some minor adjustments to the new
contract.

        1.    Por the previous Clinical Orientations, the
              maximum number of interns accommodated on each
              Ward Round was 13. Due to the increased number
              of Pharmacy Interns, this year and anticipated
              for subsequent years, it will be necessary to
              conduct three (3) orientation pej:iods each year.

        2.    I would like to receive payment for each rotation/
              orientation in two parts.

These adjustments will be incorporated in Article V and
"Statements of Services", of the contract, respectively.

Looking forward to your continued support and cooperation for
the period.

Yours sincerely,




Eugenie Brown, (Pharmacy Doctor)
CLINICAL CO-ORDINATOR

/cas
```

Appendix 4: Statement of Services for Clinical Training

<u>**Statement of Services**</u>

The Clinical component of the Pharmacy Internship Programme serves to expose pharmacy students on their practical experience to some of the clinical operations in a large hospital. The programme will be conducted on a rotation basis. Each rotation will last for approximately six (6) weeks.

The Contractor shall:

- Conduct at least two (2) rotations for each class of interns;

- make independent rounds to familiarize herself with the cases on the wards as preparation for rounds and also to be able to verify information presented by students;

- Conduct two or three ward rounds per week for interns at the same time as Medical Rounds and in conjunction with the Medical Team; (depending on hospital used and duration of Medical Rounds).

- conduct lectures and group discussions twice weekly; supervise Case Presentations to alternate with lecture sessions;

- conduct at least one seminar per rotation;

- Administer three (3) q~2zes per rotation and a final examination;

- submit to the Director of the Pharmaceutical Division a general report at the end of each rotation and progress reports on each intern.

Appendix 5: Reflections from graduates of the B.Pharm. Course of Study

My UTech Experience
By Kayon Clarke (Graduate of the Bachelor of Pharmacy class of 2001)

The anxiety that accompanies expectation can over-whelm an individual. Describing or recapturing the feeling is difficult when called upon to do some amount of reflection. September 22, 1997 marked the beginning of a lifetime of experiences at UTech that would shape the course of my professional development. I will not relay a summary of my time spent at UTech, but instead I will concisely express the lessons learnt from my experiences.

The first year is an orientation to the tasks ahead concerning the academics, working with your peers, participating in extra-curricular activities, and the dependency that occurs at the human level. The University experience is a microcosmic reflection of our society combining all the elements of specialization as well as the similarities. Learning to work with an indefatigable spirit to attain goals at an individual and at a team level defines your scope in the environment.

For those who like myself were fortunate to have lived in the campus residence had another dimension added to our learning. We lived and related to the cultural diversity that the University embraces extending to the Caribbean and the rest of the world. Here a great lesson in adaptability to a globalized world was taught in its most subtle yet powerful way. The forging of friendships and ties fostered an environment of unity by appreciating the differences amongst us. I graduated from the University of Technology, Jamaica not only with knowledge of Pharmacy and its challenges, but with an understanding of architecture, business, engineering and administrative skills that only can be garnered from the complex experiences at UTech.

The exploration of my potential throughout my four years helped in my continuously morphing definition as a cog in the system. This kept the machinery going, helped me to shoulder my responsibilities and accepted that failure is at times a much greater lesson than success, a reality in the UTech experience. Success academically is not only excellence in your career as a student, but also the appreciation of the efforts of the academics and the participation in the various organizations and activities (non-academic). This is what building the future is all bout.

Appendix 6: Reflection on Community Experience

COMMUNITY PHARMACY EXPERIENCE

By Rohan McNellie (BPharm4)

It was early Wednesday morning, and I shall never forget the shivers that ran down my spine, the tension nor my increased temperature, due to a frantically beating heart, during the orientation for the clerkship/externship programme. I was taken aback when Dr. Eugenie Brown demonstrated the kind of work required and expected of us,. It was within those moments that my inferior brain finally grasped the enormity of the situation, that I was much becoming a pharmacist, than I had ever imagine.

It was a sunny Monday morning when I arrived at Dick Kinkead, Pharmacy in Down Town Kingston. My Preceptor, Mr. R.F. Kinkead, had yet to arrive, so I introduced myself to the General Manager, Mr. G. Budal, and browsed through, what was to be, my home away from home for the next five weeks.

At precisely 8:30am a perfectly attired gentleman approached me and introduced himself as Mr. Kinkead. I must admit that I was somewhat surprised by his youthful smile and remarkable effervescence at such a golden age.

I was honored with a well guided tour of the entire store and formally introduced to the remainder of the staff. the time for business was soon at hand and I had no reservations about studying under a veteran who had been in the business longer than I had alive, over sixty years experience.

My first assignment was rather tricky, as I was unaware of what awaited me. Mr. Kinkead,after completing his morning routine of plotting the accumulative purchases on his graph and documenting the number of prescriptions done the previous day (these duties would soon revert to me), turned to me and said in his firm but friendly voice, " Professor, I have some tablets here that I take one daily in a 1 mg strength. The problem is these tablets only come in 5mg strength, what can you do for me?" I dragged in a steadying breath as he left me at the omnipotent and holy Compounding Counter and went about his usual business.

The ball was now in my court, or should I say, the prescription! I thought of a suspension (i.e. 1mg/ml) but this was an adult! After further consideration I decided to make capsules. This test,unknown to me as such, was the Doc's, as he is zealously and respectfully called, way of discovering how much I had learnt over the years. I told him how many capsules I had made and the number of 5mg tablets I had used, then he turned to me and said"you've passed, Professor. I give you a B" I then realized that Doc had conducted his own, personal orientation.

On the very first day, I found it necessary to call upon my second year dispensing skills to compound capsules, gels, suspensions, creams, ointments and not to mention, Kinkead's exclusive line of products. It was now time to ask: " *A wha' dis Fada?!*" and if that was not enough heartache, some of the prescriptions were written in the Avoirdupois system of measurement, which meant utilizing first year knowledge as well. Interestingly, on my first day I had to pull on all available resources if I were to deserve the honourary title of *Professor.*

Kinkead's Pharmacy afforded me the opportunity to exercise all the information that I had accumulated over the years.

I knew Mr. R.F. Kinkead would leave no stone unturned, when he arranged, with Major Denzil Walcot of the Salvation Army Clinic in Rae Town, for me to go over and spend three consecutive Thursdays with Dr. Bodha Rao. Nurse Pamela Maragh and Pharmacist Eurel Morrison. The experience was awesome and I realized, through Mr. Kinkead, how much of an asset a pharmacist is in innercity communities, especially in explaining drug interaction and the importance of being compliant.

I must confess, when I was first told of my new location, I was hesitant, I thought to myself that Mr. Kinkead must have a loose screw to send me to the "ghetto", but I have benefited immensely from the invaluable lessons learned.

Imagine, if you were, walking on the road and the people you pass recognize you and call you "Doc".

which reminded of what the apothecary was called then, when the druggist came down to the level of the people to give remedies and counselling to the sick and afflicted.

Mr. Kinkead displayed to me, a wealth of experience as I watched him counsel those who came in for over the counter items. I had been taught when to refer to the doctor and when to treat in Professional Practice but being around Doc you discover remedies that you would not find in any text book today.

It is always heart-stopping to stand back and observe Doc tend to each patient with gentleness and patience, never minding their background, be they homeless, destitute or Vice President of an international company.

The atmosphere at Kinkead's is warm and invitingly friendly, it's hard to tell who is the boss as teamwork is the game and it does not take you very long to become part of the family. The Pharmacist, Ms. Janet Fray, was very supportive and allowed me the opportunity to develop self-confidence, and her criticisms were greatly appreciated and did not go unnoticed. The General manager, Mr. G.W. Budal, afforded me an exclusive look into the managerial aspect of running a pharmacy and the challenges one must face in such a position. He was severely thorough when explaining to me, like a son, the procedures put in place to best operate the pharmacy in our stained economy in order to market a successful venture, and at the same time providing affordable, professional and effective service.

I would like to say a special thanks to Mr. R. F. Kinkead and staff for the once in a life time opportunity to be under their care which will no doubt shape my persona in the future, and to Ms. A. Budal for her invaluable help. Also, thanks must be extended to Dr. E. Morrison for being so kind in accommodating me.

Appendix 7: Promotional Poster BSc Pharmaceutical Technology

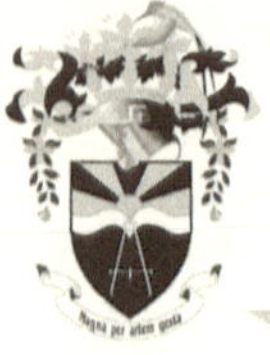

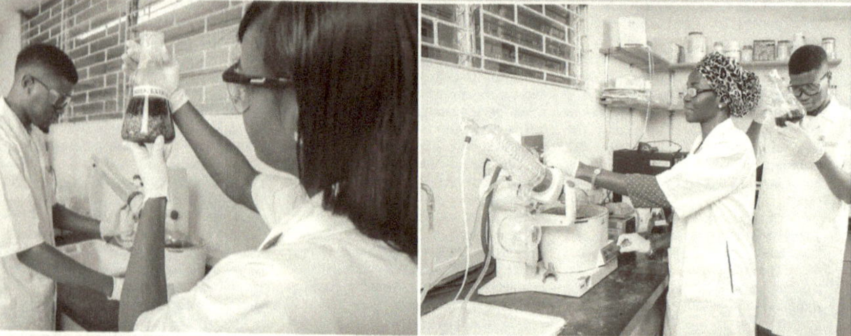

Appendix 8: Agreement between School of Pharmacy & Health Science, University of Technology, Jamaica and The Pharmacy Academic Practice Unit, University of Derby, Derby, UK.

DRAFT
November 22, 2004

COLLABORATION
Between
The School of Pharmacy & Health Science,
University of Technology, Jamaica
And
The Pharmacy Academic Practice Unit
University of Derby, Derby, UK

AGREEMENT

At the request of the administration and faculty of the University of Technology, Jamaica (herein referred to as UTech) and with the agreement of the Pharmacy Academic Practice Unit, University of Derby (hereinafter referred to as (UOD) and the University Hospital of the West Indies (hereinafter referred to as UHWI), the Pharmacy Division of the School of Pharmacy & Health Science at UTech proposes to offer the Master of Science in Clinical Pharmacy in collaboration with the University Hospital of the West Indies.

Understanding of the Parties

In anticipation of establishment of the collaboration, the Parties agree as follows:

Objectives

A.   To establish collaboration between UTech, UHWI and UOD to deliver the Master of Science in Clinical Pharmacy based on:

    a. Exchange of academic information and materials.
    b. Provision of Clinical Clerkship training at the Clinical Establishment (UHWI in this case)
    c. Provision of academic staff (Clinical Instructors, tutors) for support to the programme
    d. Support for integration of education and training in the work environment.
    e. Cooperation of all members of the Health Care team in the conduct of the programme

B.   To prepare a cadre of UTech faculty for leadership roles in the planning, implementation and delivery of future offerings of the programme.

Appendix 8: (Continued)

DRAFT
November 22, 2004

Responsibilities of the Parties

A. University of Derby agrees to :
  - Provide "learning packs" to satisfactorily offer the modules included in the programme
  - Prepare and manage assessments for students
  - Designate a UOD representative to act as programme leader and the point of contact for matters relating to the programme.

B. University of Technology, Jamaica agrees to:

  - Designate a person to act as point of contact between UTech and UOD on all matters relating to programme delivery.
  - Provide classroom facilities for delivery of tutorial sessions
  - Provide computer resource facilities, internet access, e-mail, etc
  - Provide library facilities where necessary
  - Ensure UTech faculty meets UOD requirement for provision of tutorial support
  - Promote and recruit candidates for the programme

C. University Hospital of the West Indies agrees to:
  - Provide support for the education and training in the work environment
  - Provide the clinical environment for students to gain clinical experience
  - Provide a coordinator for that aspect of the programme.

Understanding of the Parties

A. The Parties understand and agree that they are making a significant commitment to this collaborative effort. Accordingly, the Parties agree to expend their best efforts in the design, implementation, and successful continuation of the Program.

B. This agreement shall remain effective from the date of execution until the end of the agreed upon term of two to three years.

Revision or Termination of the Agreement

This agreement is subject to revision or modification by mutual consent. It is also understood that either institution may terminate this agreement at any time, although such action will only be taken after mutual consultation in order to avoid any possible inconvenience to all parties, with at least 60 days written notice to the other Party by registered mail, addressed to the Party's respective authorized representative(s), whose name(s) and title(s) appear below.

Appendix 9: MOU Letter to George Roper outlining MOU between UTech, Jamaica and University of Derby

MEMORANDUM

TO: Mr. George Roper
     Senior Vice President. Academic Affairs

FROM: Dr. Eugenie Brown-Myrie
     Head, School of Pharmacy & Health Science

C: Mrs. Carrol White
     Dean, Faculty of Health Applied Science

     Miss Delva Barnes, Faculty Administrator

     Professor Adelani Ogunrinade
     Director, Research & Graduate Studies

DATE: November 22, 2004

RE: **Collaboration between the University of Technology, Jamaica (UTech), University Hospital of the West Indies (UHWI) and the University of Derby (UOD) for the offering of a Master of Science in Clinical Pharmacy**

This serves to introduce the pilot delivery of the Master of Science in Clinical Pharmacy as a joint effort between the University of Derby and the University of Technology, Jamaica and UHWI. The programme is proposed to commence in January 2005 with a small cohort of pharmacists employed at the University Hospital of the West Indies. The Programme is work-based, and pharmacists employed in a clinical setting can pursue their studies while on the job. In this instance, the University Hospital of the West Indies will serve as the clinical facilities for this cohort of students.

The University of Derby will be responsible for the administration of the programme, will provide "learning packs" and be responsible for the granting of the awards.

The University of Technology, Jamaica, will be involved through its support in areas of facilitating tutorials, and providing clinical supervision and monitoring. The collaboration will be at minimal costs to the University of Technology.

The University of Technology, Jamaica is set to benefit from this partnership since the involvement will serve to prepare a cadre of UTech faculty for leadership roles in the planning, implementation and delivery of similar programme offerings after the expiry of

(Appendix 9 continue on next page)

Appendix 9: (Continued)

the current arrangements in 2008. If the pilot is successful, UTech will be the beneficiary of an agreement to offer the programme in the future as a UTech programme.

The details of the responsibilities of the collaborating partners are included in an accompanying draft agreement which I have prepared for consideration by all the involved parties.

Documents outlining the arrangement have previously been submitted and approved at the Faculty Board of Health & Applied Science, the Postgraduate Studies Committee and the noted at the Academic Board.

Since the University of Derby will be responsible for all aspects of the programme delivery and financial arrangements, I do not envisage any major hindrance to starting the programme in January 2005

Regards

Appendix 10: Students' Reflections on Afzal Abdool Scholarship Award

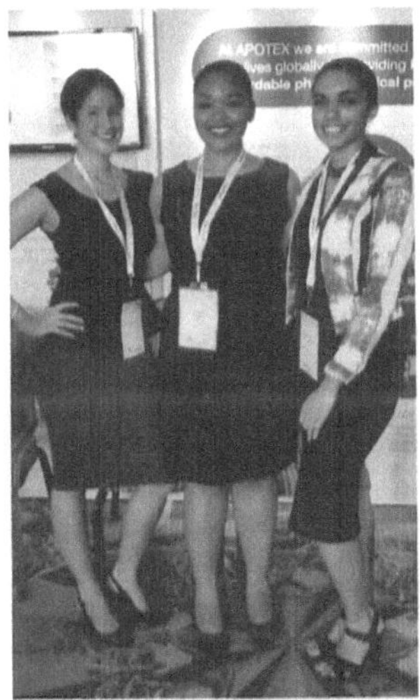

Reflections
Afzal Abdool Scholarship
Awardees 2016

We would first like to thank Dr Andrea Daly for nominating us for the Afzal Abdool Scholarship, the committee for selecting our projects, Ms Pamela Townsend and all the Caribbean Association of Pharmacists (CAP) members for warmly accommodating us. One year ago, we presented our final year research projects entitled "Knowledge and Attitudes toward Herbal vs Conventional Medicine" and "Brand Switching of Generic Metformin" at the joint CAP/PSJ Conference 2016 held in Jamaica under the theme "Pharmacists: Knowledgeable, Accessible, Promoting Health & Wellness".

The entire experience was a memorable one that has left an indelible mark on each of us. We enjoyed learning from the many different presentations and the camaraderie of everyone who attended. One major highlight of the conference for us, was being able to participate in the workshop entitled "Ethical Responsibilities in Pharmacy Practice." Our experience at the conference has offered validation of our academic choices and provided some much-needed scope for our future as pharmacists in this region. We were truly impressed by the dedication and cohesion of the CAP participants in building the profession in the Caribbean, and we remain grateful for the exposure such a platform has offered us.

Our year following the presentation of the Afzal Abdool scholarship has been one of fulfilling professional milestones. We graduated from the University of Technology with first, and upper second class honours in November 2016. Preceding this, we commenced internships and have gained valuable experience in the following areas of pharmacy:

- Community and Hospital
- Regulations
- Paediatrics

Throughout this period, we have participated in the planning and implementation of various community activities during pharmacy week. We have also gained practical learning experiences in the public health sector. We plan to continue to work and volunteer in community pharmacies to hone our soft skills in preparation for service.

By the end of this year, we expect hope to have become licenced pharmacists in Jamaica, where we will aim to be extraordinary professionals who will honour our profession and the Afzal Abdool Award. It has truly been an honour to be recognised in this way.

Sincerely,
Kristina Daley-Tomlinson, Geri Tomlin, Amanda Black

"Caribbean Pharmacists Contributing to Improved Health and Wellness of our Communities"    27

Glossary of Terms

Clerkship: A college or university coordinated practical experience conducted in patient care settings and for which academic credits are given.

Clinic Duty: An experiential training conducted within a College Community pharmacy located on a college or university campus.

Continuing Education (CE): Formal lectures, courses, seminars, webinars, or any other similar type of educational program designed to educate an individual and give him or her further skills or knowledge to be applied in his or her line of work. These programs are intended to educate persons on new advancements, or to build upon a person's expertise in a given field. These may be optional for some trades, but in other circumstances can be required to maintain status, certification, or licensure.

Continuing Professional Development (CPD): A combination of different approaches, ideas and techniques that will assist a professional in managing his/her own learning and growth. It involves each individual assessing his/her educational needs, planning and carrying out learning, reviewing the learning outcomes and activities, implementing the knowledge gained in practice, reflecting on the knowledge gained and identifying additional needs.

Course of Study: A structured academic programme that can result in achievements such as certificates or degrees.

Curriculum: A course of study in one subject at a school or college. It is also described as any programme or plan of activities.

Externship: A college or university coordinated practical experience conducted in pharmacies and for which academic credits are awarded

Internship: Vocational training of Pharmacy Interns in approved hospitals, community pharmacies or other approved institutions for a period of twelve months as a prerequisite for registration as Pharmacists.

Module: A standardized or self-contained segment that with other such segments constitutes an educational course or training program (http://www.businessdictionary.com/definition/module.html)

Programme: A collection or series of courses that lead to a degree, certificate, or transfer to another institution of higher éducation

Syllabus: An outline or other brief statement of the main points of a discourse, the subjects of a course of lectures, the contents of a curriculum

References

Accreditation Council for Pharmacy Education – ACPE. (2007). Accreditation Council for Pharmacy Education Definition of Continuing Education for the Profession of Pharmacy. Retrieved from https://.acpe-accredit.org/pdf/Definition of CE.pdf

Accreditation Council for Pharmacy Education – ACPE. (2014). Continuing Professional Development (online) Education for the Profession of Pharmacy. Retrieved from https://www.acpeaccreditorg/pharmacists/CPDasp.

Adebayo, S., Brown Myrie, E. (2005–2006). Research Development Fund Final Report. University of Technology, Jamaica Kingston, Jamaica: Author.

Allen, G. (1990, January–March). *The Pharmacy Newsletter*, 2 (1), 3.

Allen Young, E.G. (1995, June). Commonwealth Pharmacy Day Message, Commonwealth Pharmaceutical Association Bulletin.

Allen Young, G. (1999, March–June). CPA Representative Message. Common Waves, 2 (2), 1–2.

Bachelor of Pharmacy Course of Study Curriculum. (1996). University of Technology, Jamaica, Kingston, Jamaica: Author.

Bailey, R. (2005, June). President's Report, *Pharmaceutical Society of Jamaica Retreat magazine*, 3.

Bell, J. (1999, July–August). President's Address, Commonwealth Pharmaceutical Association (CPA). Common Waves, 2(3), 2.

Bromfield, L. (2010, June). Continuing Education and Training Committee Chair's Report, Pharmaceutical Society of Jamaica. Kingston, Jamaica.

Brown, E. (1980). *Introduction to Pharmacy* [Lecture Notes]. Kingston, Jamaica.

Brown, E. (1989). Pharmacy Diploma and Degree Programs in the Caribbean. Joint Conference of the Commonwealth Pharmaceutical Association (Americas Region) and the Caribbean Association of Pharmacists. Ottawa, Canada.

Brown, E. (1999, July/August). New role for the pharmacist in the 21st century. *Common Waves*, 2(3), 4.

Canadian Council for Accreditation of Pharmacy Programs. (2014). Retrieved from https://www.acpe-accredit.org/international-services-program/

Canadian Society of Hospital Pharmacists Statement. (1995). Retrieved from https://www.cshp.ca/

CCAPP Accreditation Standards for Canadian First Professional Degree in Pharmacy Programs. (2018). Retrieved August 2, 2108 from http://ccapp-accredit.ca/wp-content/uploads/2016/01/Accreditation-Standards-for-Canadian-First-Professional-Degree-in-Pharmacy-Programs.pdf.

Cox, S. (2016). Electronic Prescribing Service Providers' Guidelines, Pharmacy Council of Jamaica. (Unpublished data). Kingston, Jamaica.

Cross, C.J., Tofade, T. (2014). Continuing professional development/continuing education in Pharmacy: Global Report. International Pharmaceutical Federation (FIP). The Hague, The Netherlands.

Doctor of Pharmacy (PharmD) Programme Curriculum (2009). University of Technology, Jamaica: Kingston, Jamaica: Author.

Doctor of Pharmacy (PharmD) Programme Accreditation. Retrieved August 2, 2018 from https://www.acpe-accredit.org/pharmd-program-accreditation/.

Donyai, P., Herbert, RZ., Denicolo, P.M., & Alexander, A.M. (2011) British Pharmacy professionals' beliefs and participation in continuing professional development: a review of the literature. *International Journal of Pharmacy Practice*, 19(5): 290–317.

Draft Reciprocal Agreement (2013), Kingston, Jamaica.

Driesen, A., Leemans, L., Baert, H., & Laekerman, G. (2005). Flemish community pharmacists' motivation and views relating to continuing education. *Pharmacy World and Science*, 27(6): 447–52.

Driesen, A., Verbeke, K., Simoens, S., & Laekerman, G. (2007) International trends in lifelong learning for pharmacists. *American Journal of Pharmacy Education*, Jun 25; 71(3): 52.

Dunn, N. (2016, July). Chairman's Message, Pharmacy Council of Jamaica. Conference Magazine Pharmaceutical Society of Jamaica, 10. Ellis, P (2009)

FIP Centennial Congress Programme (2012). The FIP Centennial Improving health through responsible medicines use. Retrieved from https://www.fip.org/files/congress/FIP.2012_Final Programme_LA_v7.pdf.

FIP Global Report (2014). Together we are stronger. Retrieved from https://www.fip.org/files/fip/2015-Annual_report_for_2014_spread.pdf.

Forbes, G. (2005, June). Message from the Chairman Pharmacy Council of Jamaica. Pharmaceutical Society of Jamaica, *Retreat Magazine*, page 9.

Higby, G.J. (2005). *Evolution of Pharmacy. In Remington: The Science and Practice of Pharmacy*. (21st ed., pp. 7–19) Philadephia, PA: Lippincott Williams & Wilkins.

Gray, CA; Woolery, L. (2005, June). Spotlight on the life of Mr Van Gladstone Knight. Pharmaceutical Society of Jamaica, *Retreat Magazine*, June 24–26, 2005, 26–27.

Gray, CA. (n.d). The History of Pharmacy in Jamaica. (Unpublished Workshop Presentation). Kingston, Jamaica.

Grizzle, E. (1994, July). Guidance on continuing education participation. Pharmaceutical Society of Jamaica.

Grizzle, E. (1999, January–February). New role for the Pharmacist in the 21st Century. *Common Waves*, 2(1), 3.

Grizzle, E. (2003, March–April). New business opportunities-sports medicine: Taking care of the medication needs of the Caribbean's elite athletes. Caribbean Pharmacy News, 5(2), 6–14.

Hall, J (2003). *Kingston Public Hospital: The High Seat of Medicine in Jamaica.* Pelican Publishers, Limited. Eden Gardens, Kingston, Jamaica.

Hanson, AL., Bruskiewitz, R.H., & Demuth, J.E. (2007, August 15). Pharmacists' perceptions of facilitators and barriers to lifelong learning. *American Journal of Pharmacy Education*, 71(4), 67.

Harris H. (2004, June) Pharmacy Management: A change to come. Pharmaceutical Society of Jamaica, *Retreat Magazine*, 17.

Haughton, S. (2018). Pharmacy in Jamaica: A personal perspective. *Pharmaceutical Society of Jamaica, Conference Magazine*, 24–31.

History and Heritage, University of Manchester. Retrieved from https://www.bmh.manchester.ac.uk/about/history-heritage.

Ibrahim, M. (2012, April). Assessment of Egyptian pharmacists' attitude, behaviors, and preferences related to continuing education. International Journal of Clinical Pharmacy, 34(2), 358–63.

International Pharmaceutical Federation- FIP (2002). FIP Statement of Professional Standards Continuing Professional Development. The Hague, The Netherlands. International Pharmaceutical Federation (online) Retrieved from https://www.fip.org/file/1544.

Johnson-Reid, Y. (2002). UHWI Certificate Pharmacy Technician Training Curriculum (Unpublished work, Kingston, Jamaica.

Jones, A. (2017, June). President's Report. Pharmaceutical Society of Jamaica, *Conference Magazine*, 4.

Koshman S.L., Blais J. (2011, March). What is Pharmacy Research? *Can J Hosp Pharm.* 64(2), 154–5.

Lowe, H.I.C. (1973). Trends in Pharmaceutical Education: A Review on Jamaica. Unpublished work, Kingston, Jamaica.

Moncrieffe, S. (2014). Memorandum to Staff, College of Health Sciences, University of Technology, Jamaica.

Manual for Pharmacy Internship. (2018). Publication of the Pharmacy Council of Jamaica. Kingston, Jamaica: Author.

Marotta, R. (2017). How One Student Is Improving Patient Health and the Pharmacy Profession. Pharmacy Times, Feb. 2017. Retrieved from https://www.pharmacytimes.com/publications/issue/2017/february2017/how-one-student-is-improving-patient-health-and-the-pharmacy-profession.

Memorandum of Agreement (MOA) between College of Arts, Science and Technology (CAST), Jamaica and the School of Community and Allied Health, University of Alabama at Birmingham, (SCAH/UAB). (1984) (Unpublished data). Kingston, Jamaica: Author.

Pan American Health Organisation (2013). (Unpublished, Preliminary Meeting Notes). Kingston, Jamaica: Author

PCJ Update (2007, August). Publication of the Pharmacy Council of Jamaica. 5(1) 2.

PCJ Update (2010, June,). Publication of the Pharmacy Council of Jamaica. 8(1), 3.

PHACE '94: (1994, February). For Advancement in Pharmacy Knowledge. *PSJ Annual Pharmacy Magazine*, 1, 35.

Pharmaceutical Society of Jamaica/Caribbean Association of Pharmacists. (2016). Conference Magazine, Kingston, Jamaica: Author.

Pharmaceutical Society of Jamaica. (2010). Second Vice President's Report 2009/10. Kingston, Jamaica: Author.

Policy on External Examiners. (2017/2018). *Undergraduate Student Handbook*. Student Services and Registry, University of Technology, Jamaica. Kingston, Jamaica.

Policy on Advisory Committees. (2008). University of Technology, Jamaica. Kingston, Jamaica: Author.

Reid, Y. (2013). The History of Pharmacy in Jamaica (Unpublished Work). Kingston, Jamaica.

Reid Y. (2017). *Caribbean Association of Pharmacists: Surveying the Past; Seizing the Future*. In Print.

Roper, G. (1990). C.A.S.T. '89–'90: Excellence against all odds. *Student's Union Yearbook*. Kingston, Jamaica: Author.

Roper, G., & Sangster, A.W. (1989). The development of a Health Sciences Post Diploma Degree Programme at the College of Arts, Science & Technology. New Developments in Education. Unpublished work. Kingston, Jamaica.

Sangster, A. (2010). *The Making of a University: From CAST to UTech. Kingston, Jamaica*: Ian Randle Publishers.

Social Impact/Activism. ACS; Chemistry for life. Retrieved from https://www.acs.org/content/acs/en/careers/college-to-career/chemistry-careers/social-impact.html

Strein, G.W., Mallman, J.C. (1975). A teaching program in clinical pharmacy in Jamaica. Project HOPE: The People to People Health Foundation, Inc., Washington, DC.

UTech Broadcaster (2013) First Cohort of Online Pharmacy Students complete didactic studies. Kingston, Jamaica. Author.

University of Technology, Jamaica, Summary of Programmes (2012/2013). Kingston, Jamaica: Author.

University of Technology, Jamaica & The College of the Bahamas Franchise Agreement (2008). Kingston, Jamaica: Author.

University of Technology, Jamaica & University of Derby Agreement (2004), Kingston, Jamaica: Author.

University Council of Jamaica (2017, October). *Manual for the Visiting Team.* Kingston, Jamaica.

University of the West Indies, Mona. (2016). Doctor of Pharmacy Curriculum. Kingston, Jamaica

UTAPS Mortar & Pestle (1999–2000). Scholarship Advertisement, Front inside Cover. Kingston, Jamaica.

Vaughan, LR. (1990, September–December). Of this and that in the Pharmaceutical Society of Jamaica. *Pharmacy Newsletter* 2(2), 2–3, 11.

Wallace, L. (2005, November). Pharmacy Council of Jamaica (PCJ) Update 3(1), 2.

Wilbur, K. (2010, August). Continuing professional pharmacy development needs assessment of Qatar pharmacists. *International Journal of Pharmacy Practice* (4), 236–41.

Woolery, L. (1999, Aug/Sep). My word is my bond. *Caribbean Pharmacy News,* 1(4), 22, 24.

Woolery, L. (2000, July/Aug). Build the Future on the Fires of the Past. *Caribbean Pharmacy News,* 2(4) 20.

Woolery, L. (2008, June). Chairman's Message, Pharmacy Council of Jamaica. Pharmaceutical Society of Jamaica, *Conference Magazine*, page 11.

Woolery, L. (2009, June). Career paths in pharmacy. *PCJ Update,* 7(1), 1, 3

Index